Nutritional Healing

Avicenna Institute Course

By Kristie Karima Burns, MH, ND, Ph.D.

ISBN 978-1-304-17923-4
Text Copyright © 2013 by Kristie Karima Burns, MH, ND, Ph.D.
All rights reserved. Published by BEarth Publishing
Library of Congress Cataloging-in-Publication Data available.
Printed in the U.S.A
First Edition, August 1997
Second Edition, December 2009
Third Edition, June 2013

The Avicenna Institute Naturopathic Healing Classes
www.TheAvicennaInstitute.com

101 Nutritional Healing
201 Herbal Preparations
202 Herbal First Aid
203 Herbs for Women
204 Herbal Healing
301 Aromatherapy
401 Reflexology
501 Iridology
502 Advanced Iridology
601 Homeopathy Case Taking
602 Homeopathic Remedies
701 Consultations
801 Typology

101: Nutritional Healing

This *unit* stands alone as a certification class in nutritional healing. It is also the first *unit* in the Naturopathic Healing Course at www.TheAvicennaInstitute.com. This *unit,* like all *units* in the course is divided into *sections.* Each section may have several topics and may or may not have a quiz after it. If you are enrolled as a full student please take the quiz or do the assignment after each section (if there is one) and send it to: exams@TheBEarthInstitute.com . If you are an audit student you may do the assignments and quizzes for your own benefit. However, you will not be able to have them marked and commented on by an instructor. If you have trouble with this process please use the FAQs page at www.TheBEarthInstitute.com to contact the instructor.

When you send the quiz to your instructor and s/he corrects it you get credit for the quiz. It may take up to a month for instructors to correct quizzes, however, so once you turn in your assignment, please go to the next section and complete as many assignments or quizzes as you want to. There is no set order to the lessons because you work at your own pace. We are always improving these courses to better them, make them easier to use, and be more comprehensive in each course. Some of these courses include video and MP3 as well as these written lessons. However, these *written* lessons are what you will be tested on. The MP3s and videos are supplements to make your own learning process more enjoyable and efficient. However, they do not contain extra information or information you will be tested on. If there is an idea you have about a course please let us know. These are courses that evolve just as holistic medicine evolves in understanding, theory, practice, acceptance, and teaching. As technology expands our universe these courses will use this advance to help teach more effectively these ideas. However, also keep in mind that the content of these courses does not change. The courses may be re-formatted and we may add videos and MP3s, however, this does not affect your previous work in the course. If materials are updated or change you do not need to re-do any assignments or quizzes.

General Information

Nutritional Healing 101 consists of the lectures and writings in this book. Please read and study these. There will be a series of quizzes and/or essays after each section or set of sections. Do not worry if there is a section without a quiz. Some sections do not have quizzes. After you have finished reading each section please take the quiz for that section and send it to exams@TheBEarthInstitute.com. You will be sent a certificate of completion after each three units you complete. You may take the units in any order and you may choose to take one, two, three or even all of the units. Once you complete three units you need to make a "request for certificates" to the FAQs/Contact Us page with the following information: (1) the name you want on the certificate, (2) your current address and (3) the certificates requested.

Goals of this Unit

To show the student how nutrition makes a key difference in their health. This unit will not just teach the student about "good" and "bad" foods. This is a useless way of looking at foods. Rather, this unit will teach the student how to choose the best foods according to the season, their body type, their blood type, moderation rules and other theories. This unit will teach the student that there is a lot more to food than "good" and "bad". This unit will also explore what "natural foods" really are and how we benefit from nature.

Additional Recommended Texts for this Unit

These are not required readings. These are readings that other students, practitioners and clients have found useful over the past few years. These readings may also be part of your extra reading list if you choose to upgrade your class to a Bachelor's or Master's degree.

"The Detox Box" by Nic Rowley and Kirsten Hartwig includes massage instructions and three detoxifying pure essential oils as well as recipes for a seven day fast.

"Complete Guide to Vitamins, Minerals & Supplements" by H. Winter Griffith, M.D.

"Prescription for Nutritional Healing" Balch, Phyllis and Balch, Dr. James Avery Press. 2003.

"Handbook of Phytochemical Constituents of GRAS Herbs and Other Economic Plants" Duke, J. A. CRC Press. Boca Raton, FL, 1992.

"Heinerman's Encyclopedia of Nature's Vitamins and Minerals." Heinerman, John. Prentice Hall: New Jersey. 1998.

"The New Orthomolecular Nutrition." Hoffer, Abram and Pauling, Linus Keats Publishing: New Canaan, 1995.

"New Foods for Healing." Yeager, Selene. Rodale Press: Pennsylvania. 1998.

Required Reading for this Unit

These readings are all contained in this book.

Section One: Nutritional Healing: Overview
"Living Closer to Nature and Its Maker: The Twelve Principals of Healing" by Kristie Karima Burns, Mh, ND

Section Two: Nutritional Healing: Modern Nutritional Dangers
Articles written by Kristie Karima Burns, Mh, ND, on the following topics: acidic food, alcohol, aluminum, aspartame and MSG, chlorine and fluoride, coffee, colloidal silver, cow's milk, dietary supplements and vitamins excess, bread and carbohydrate addiction, soda pop, sodium laurel sulfate and other chemicals, and tobacco.

Section Three: Nutritional Healing: The Four Humors and Nutrition
"The History and Theory of Temperament in Islamic Medicine." by Kristie Karima Burns, Mh, ND
"The Three Schools of Greek Medicine." by Kristie Karima Burns, Mh, ND
"The History of Temperament and Temperament Theory in all World Religions and Systems." by Kristie Karima Burns, Mh, ND
"The Physical Characteristics of Temperament." by Kristie Karima Burns, Mh, ND *"Temperament and Depression."* by Kristie Karima Burns, Mh, ND
"Humeral Properties of Foods and Herbs" by Kristie Karima Burns, Mh, ND
Word Comparison Chart of The Four Humors in Healing, Nutrition and Personality by Kristie Karima Burns, Mh, ND

Section Four: Nutritional Healing: Diets for Healing
Diets for healing edited and revised by Kristie Karima Burns, Mh, ND: Anti-Hypoglycemic, Balancing Diet /Anti-Acid, Blood Building Diet, Candida Diet, Detox Fast-Tibb, Detox Warning, Green Drink Fast, Haas Detox, High Phosphorus, LOW Carb Diet, Non-toxic diet (basic,) Rotation Diet and Universal Parasite Cleanse.

Section Five: Nutritional Healing: Vitamins for Healing
"Nutritional Healing with Supplements: Is it Possible?" by Kristie Karima Burns, Mh, ND

Section Six: Nutritional Healing: The Kitchen Pharmacy
"The Kitchen Pharmacy" by Kristie Karima Burns, Mh, ND
The Four Types Chart

~Section One: Nutritional Healing Overview~

The Twelve Principles of Health
by Kristie Karima Burns, Mh, ND

Note: The point of this lecture is not to show that religion is the basis of nutrition. It is meant to show how important nutrition is to the three major world religions and to correlate that to modern science. Whatever spiritual or religious beliefs you have this article will not only help teach you the twelve principles of health but also their place in history and in many cultures of the world. This integration of thought becomes especially important when working with friends, family and clients. This also provides a guide for you to apply this integration to other cultural morals and values you may encounter in friends, family and clients.

Dr. E. S. Rogers, in his text, Human Ecology and Health says, *"One has little difficulty in distinguishing between life and death, but the distinction between illness and health is not as easy."*[1]

How *can* it be easy? In the supermarket one is bombarded with sugar-laden, processed & packaged foods marked "wholesome" while numerous studies show that these products are far from wholesome. Simultaneously we are flooded with magazine advertisements that promise us good health in a bottle of supplements and yet our health care provider tells us that taking a supplement cannot solve all of our problems. We are also fed a media overdose of "medical information" that claims eggs and various other foods are unhealthy, only to retract their statements ten years later. Through the media we are taught that illness is something bad we must crush with pills and health is something only awarded to those who buy expensive exercise equipment and *specially packaged* herbal supplements. With all the conflicting information, how can a person find their way in today's world?

The answer is a more straightforward than it seems. Hundreds of organizations are looking for cures for diseases, thousands of companies are marketing supplements and millions of varieties of "healthy" foods go in and out of fashion. However, the one source you can consult to help you rise above all the clutter is your religion, which will advise you to live closer to nature and its maker. Although the concept of living closer to nature and its maker sounds simple, applying it to everyday life is not as clear. It takes faith, dedication and most of all knowledge to be able to apply the principals of healthy living through a natural and spiritual lifestyle. Once you understand the basic principles you can apply them to all aspects of your life, realize their interrelations and enjoy a healthy physical and spiritual life.

There are twelve main categories or *principals* of health. The cornerstone of the twelve basic principles of health is faith. The ten building blocks of health are optimism and a happy outlook on life, whole foods, real foods, raw foods, appropriate foods, exercise, pure water, pure air, using natural therapies and substances to heal, and self-awareness. The "glue" that holds all these together, and the final, twelfth principal is knowledge.

Defining faith as the cornerstone of health is difficult. For just as *Dr. Rogers* pointed out in his statement, *"the distinction between health and illness is not as clear as the distinction between life and death"*, we can also say the same of our relationship with God in these categories. Most people agree that we have a Maker that gave us life, and those same people (even if it is on their deathbed) hope to pass from death to an afterlife in heaven. But their relationship to God in the interim leads them down endless pathways. However, in all world religions from the Hindu to Navaho's there is a distinct link between one's religious duties and one's health. Yet, rather than try to cover all religions, in this dissertation, I have chosen to focus on three major world religions as defined by the World Book Encyclopedia 1999 Edition - Christianity, Islam and Judaism. This dissertation in no way condones or negates any religion mentioned but merely compares their views on health. This is not a religious argument or dissertation, it is a guideline for health using examples from various scriptures. In the past ten years there have been an increasing number of Christian books that focus on the subject of herbs and religion or vegetarianism and religion. This dissertation aims to illustrate that not only are Christian's linked to God by healthy living, but that this bond is *universal* and people of all religions feel that same bond. So how does healthy living relate to faith?

As a matter of fact, they are interrelated. The well-respected homeopath, Dr. Rocine believed that sensory, intellectual and spiritual experiences are as necessary to feed the mind, soul and spirit as food is necessary for the health of the body. He believed that poor food habits that result in nutrient deficiencies in the brain could lead to mental disease and mild to bizarre misbehavior. So could long-term exposure to an environment stripped of beauty, meaning and hope.[2] He demonstrated and observed in his many years as a homeopath that this lack of faith (which he defined as beauty, meaning and hope) could cause disease just as easily as a lack of nutrients in the body. The reverse is also true. Not only can a lack of faith cause disease, but disease can also effect one's faith. Dr. Bernard Jensen stated in his book The Chemistry of Man that, *"Whole foods inspire wholeness and wellness in a person"*[3]. Jacqueline Krohn, in her book, The Whole Way to Allergy Relief and Prevention states that, *"There is a crucial relationship between good health and your emotional, mental and spiritual condition"*[4]. So not only does faith have something to do with health, but the two are interdependent and inseparable.

Our sense of duty to God also plays a big role in our view on health. In all three of the primary world religions respect for the body is mentioned in all the holy books of those religions. Various quotes are included in the text of this dissertation.

We can use this cornerstone of faith to help us build the ten building blocks of health by using our religious instructions as a guide & map to our health instead of the fickle media of ads, TV and "medical reports". The former is eternal wisdom from God and will serve us well in our quest for health, while the latter is fabricated from ever changing ideas created largely around the goal of achieving earthly pleasures and gaining wealth or fame.

The Second Building Block of Health: Mental Calm and a Positive Outlook

Examples of the virtues of a positive mental attitude, perseverance and optimism in regard to adversity:

- *"A cheerful heart is a good medicine, but a downcast spirit dries up the bones."* (Proverbs 19:22: Bible)
- *"Pleasant words are like a honeycomb, sweetness to the soul and health to the body."* (Proverbs. 16:24 :Bible)
- *"Give Glad tidings to those who exercise patience when struck with adversity and say, 'indeed we belong to God and to him is our return' such ones receive blessings and Mercy of their lord, and such are the guided ones"* (Koran 2:155)
- *"And now it came to pass that the burdens which were laid upon Alma and his brethren were made light; yea, the Lord did strengthen them that they could bear up their burdens with ease, and they did submit cheerfully and with patience to all the will of the Lord."[5]* (Book of Mormon Mosiah 24:15)

At one of the most critical junctures of Jewish history, with Assyrian King Sennacherib's vast army closing in on Jerusalem, Hezekiah King of Judah suddenly fell mortally ill. His entire body was covered with horrible sores. The prophet Isaiah came to him and said,

- *"Thus says the Lord: Set your house in order, for you will die and not live"* (Isaiah 38:1; Kings II, 20:1)

With God's prophet telling him to make his will and prepare to die, a lesser man might have given up the fight. Not Hezekiah. He had a tradition from his ancestor, King David:

- *"Even if a sharp sword is pressing on your neck, don't despair of pleading for God's mercy"* (Berakhot 10a*). Hezekiah turned his face to the wall and prayed: "Remember now, O God, I beseech You, how I've walked before You in truth and with a whole heart: I did what is good in Your eyes. Hezekiah wept bitterly."* (Jewish)[6]
- *"The LORD is my shepherd; I shall not want. He maketh me to lie down in green pastures: he leadeth me beside the still waters. He restoreth my soul: he leadeth me in the paths of righteousness for his name's sake. Yea, though I walk through the valley of the shadow of death, I will fear no evil: for thou art with me; thy rod and thy staff they comfort me. Thou preparest a table before me in the presence of mine enemies: thou anointest my head with oil; my cup runneth over. Surely goodness and mercy shall follow me all the days of my life: and I will dwell in the house of the LORD for ever."* (Bible: Psalms 23)
- *King Solomon said, "On a good day, enjoy! And on a bad day, you must look"* (Ecclesiastes 7:14).

The second building block of health is to be positive and not negative about life. To be thankful for what we have, to be relaxed, calm and optimistic. Bernard Jensen, in his book, The Science and Practice of Iridology says, " The doctor of the new day will recognize that a man's most important workshop is not the physical body but the mind that controls it".[7] Dr. Ted M. Morter, in his book Your Health...Your Choice confirms this when he says that "negative thoughts are the number one acid producer in the body...because your body reacts to negative mental and emotional stress brought about by thought the same way it reacts to 'real' threats of physical harm."[8]   In fact, of all the patients who consult outpatient clinical facilities in the United States, an astounding seventy percent are found to have no organic basis for their complaint.[9]

Seventy percent is an overwhelming figure. However, although statistically there is no obvious organic source of many patients' complaints, there is actually a physical basis for this phenomenon. Ever since Freud popularized the idea of psychoanalysis, people have been looking to the mental realm to solve their problems, forgetting all the while that you cannot separate the mental realm (the mind) from the physical realm (the body). For the mind *is* in the brain and the brain is an organ, like all other organs, and it feeds on the same nutrient pool the other organs feed on and is susceptible to all of the same problems (inflammation, tumors, pain, etc...). Ultimately, the brain is just a part of our body like the rest of us. The brain is, in fact, completely dependent on the body. It requires sugar and cannot even develop energy from potassium and fats as other tissues can. Because of this the brain is the first organ to suffer from lack of blood sugar and reacts most severely.[10]   Freud himself even said that psychoanalysis was not suitable for such diseases as schizophrenia and postulated that the cause eventually would be found to be biochemical.[11]

So if we keep in mind that the brain is an organ and that it works in harmony with the other organs and feeds from the same bloodstream as the other organs we can understand how various mental events could affect us physically. For example, simply using our brain to *think* can burn up nutrients in our system, particularly phosphorus. As the brain uses a lot of phosphorus to function, using the brain heavily can burn up excess phosphorus and cause us to have symptoms of a phosphorus deficiency.[12] To emphasize this relationship you can also find that the reverse is true. People who have high intellectual capacity such as psychic perceptions, idealistic tendencies and humanitarianism usually have high levels of phosphorus in their system. [13]

But phosphorus is not the only nutrient that can be depleted by mental stress. The emotions, which are mostly handled by the thyroid gland can cause a deficiency of iodine if strong emotions cause the thyroid to work overtime.[14]   Even hypoglycemia can be caused by excitement. When a person sees something exciting it stimulates the adrenal cortex through the lens of the eye and causes an increase in blood sugar. This in turn stimulates the pancreas to secrete insulin into the blood and the person becomes tired or weak with the lowered blood sugar levels.[15] Stress itself, from a high-tension job, move or divorce can cause a loss of potassium and sodium in the body because stress effects the adrenal glands which create more of a need for these minerals.

The best way to keep one's mind from controlling one's matter, though, is simply to be aware of what mental capacities one is using and be aware of what it may be doing to the body. For instance, if a person is up late studying every night, they may want to concentrate on eating phosphorus rich foods and foods that help maintain their intake of phosphorus. If a person is moving or traveling they may want to make sure they increase their intake of foods high in potassium and sodium, as well as vitamin B complex. On the other hand, if humanity completely ignores that fact that the mind can control the health of the body, then they are missing an important detail in the picture of personal health. The relationship is so strong, in fact, that Anne Frohm, in her book The Cancer Battle Plan noticed that " *Those who tend towards passive acceptance of what they've been told is their inevitable fate (and play the role of the victim)...usually die right on schedule*"[16]. To make matters even more complicated some therapists advise that you should not even eat at all while you are upset, as it impairs the digestive process altogether. [17]

Not surprisingly, this relationship goes both ways. Not only does the mind control the health of the body, but the health of the body also can control the mind. In the wake of many recent publicly violent crimes, a number of health care professionals have come out and blamed the highly processed and nutrient deficient American diet as one of the villains. This is not a new idea at all. One study of juvenile delinquents showed that when the boys at the juvenile home were given a diet of whole grains and healthy food their behavior disorders literally vanished. When they returned to their white bread regime, the problems started up again. [18] This problem has become so obvious in some cases that lawyers are worried that these new findings may create a rash of people blaming their food for their behavior. They are calling this new "food-controlling-behavior" excuse "the Twinkie Defense". Boston Red Socks shortstop Stan Paus was sent to a mental hospital, drugged, given electric shock and driven to the edge of suicide because the doctors could not recognize the symptoms of low blood sugar - hypoglycemia. After beginning a strict diet he was back to normal in two months. [19]

Yet, this is not just a matter of listing a few isolated cases. The relationship is so strong between the nutrients in the body and the mind that when animals lack magnesium, they refuse to nurse their young. [20] One wonders if perhaps this also has anything to do with the present nutrient- deficient society and its preference of bottle-feeding over breastfeeding. Bernard Jensen even theorizes that *"We are going to find that divorces are, to a great extent, influenced by the foods we eat. Lifeless foods produce lifeless marriages where magnetic current fails to flow between partners."*[21]

Taking the mind and body interrelationship one step farther is the therapy of biofeedback, which bases its system on the proof that the conscious mind can command the unconscious to restore bodily functions to normal.[22] Dr. Irving Oyle, in his book, The Healing Mind, found that the two factors of trust and will were two of the greatest factors in whether a patient would be healed or not, no matter which kind of therapy they used. In all cases the patient simply needed to have complete faith in the method and person he was using and also to have a will to live. Dr. Oyle witnessed more than one case of a patient who died simply because they wanted to or did not get well because they had no faith in the person helping them. [23]

The Third Building Block of Health: Eat Whole Foods

Examples in Scriptures of the Virtues of Whole Foods:

- *"Ye People, eat of what is on earth, lawful and wholesome"* (Koran 2:168)
- *"If the patient can be treated through diet alone he should not be treated with medicines. If it is impossible to control the illness without medications, the first choice should be medicines that are nourishing and foods that have medicinal properties."* *Rambam* (Rabbi Moshe Ben Maimon, Maimonides, 1135-1204)(2:21-22) (Jewish)
- *"He causeth the grass to grow for the cattle, and herb for the service of man: that he may bring forth food out of the earth"* (Bible:Psalms 104:14)
- *"Much food is in the tillage of the poor (the whole food): but there is that is destroyed for want of judgment."* (Bible:Proverbs 13:23)
- *"And again, verily I say unto you, all wholesome herbs God hath ordained for the constitution, nature, and use of man—"* [24](Doctrine & Covenants 89:10)

The third rule of health is to eat whole foods. Many people have a hard time understanding what a "whole" food is. In 1940 about 80% of the nation consumed whole foods. Today only 25% do.[25] Obviously, we all need a refresher course in whole foods. A whole food is merely a food that retains its original constituents. An apple is a whole food and applesauce made from fresh apples at home in a grinder is a whole food but applesauce ground and cooked by machines and separated to create a better texture and then supplemented with sugar and color is not a whole food. Wheat Berries are a whole food. Flour made from pure ground wheat berries is a whole food, but flour made by separating the bran and germ and then bleaching the final product (white flour) is not a whole food. Even some popular "health food" items fall in the category of processed partial foods (and not whole). This list includes rice cakes, granola bars, pretzels, turkey and tofu hot dogs, whole grain cereals and frozen juices. These so called "health foods" are only a tiny fraction more nutritious and less dangerous than their mainstream processed counterparts. So why is it so important to eat the whole food? Why isn't just part of the food good enough?

Because grains, vegetables and fruits, the way we find them in nature, contain all the nutrients we need to thrive as human beings, and the more we change them from their original state, the less gain we get from them. More than one hundred years ago when vitamin research began, man started to think that they could change food into a more desirable substance (white flour) and then simply "enrich" back in the vitamins and minerals they took out. Abram Hoffer, MD, says, *"This is the same as being held up at gunpoint on a dark street* *and ordered to strip naked. The thief takes your clothes and valuables, notices your shivering embarrassment and then returns your underwear and $1.50 to take the bus home. Do you then feel enriched?"*[26] With new vitamins and minerals being discovered every year, it is becoming increasingly obvious that mother nature is way ahead of us and we are not even close to knowing all of the secrets of what makes food good for us, let alone being able to duplicate that process in a laboratory. As Bernard Jensen says, "Natural foods contain all the vitamins that have been and will be discovered"[27] This apparent fact should also make it obvious to people that the only way to *guarantee* you are getting all your nutrients is to get them from whole foods. To use any other method to build health, is merely an educated guess.

It does not make sense to eat devitalized foods for our entire life and then spend time and money buying vitamins, taking supplements and following various health programs. Why don't we just eat the whole food from the very beginning? However, just eating whole grains and fresh produce is not enough. We are so accustomed to throwing out parts of our foods or buying our foods with missing parts, some of us do not even know what a whole food looks like. For instance, watermelon is a whole food, but not if you spit out the seeds. The seeds have been shown to aid in such conditions as hypertension, nephritis and kidney disturbances. Nuts are also a whole food, but not if you buy them shelled. Once the nut leaves the shell, the oils (high in manganese) have been disintegrated or oxidized.[28] Another example is Pumpkins. Many people are in the habit of scooping out the seeds in their squash or pumpkin and then cooking and eating the nutritious pumpkin. However, the seeds also have benefits, especially to the prostate gland and heart, and are meant to be eaten as well.

We have already established that whole foods are superior to processed foods, but some people may still argue that that is not a good enough reason for them to stop eating processed foods. Others say, *"So what? Processed foods are not as good, but they won't kill me."* Certainly they will not kill a person as fast as processed foods with chemicals, sugars and colorings added, but they will eventually chip away at their health. For processed foods are not just lacking in nutrients, *they also take nutrients from the system.*

First of all, processed foods do not have enough vitamins and minerals to help in their own assimilation. An analysis of the ascorbic acid content of potatoes revealed a 91.4% loss from the raw potato after harvest to the reconstituted flakes.[29] Pasta, for instance, does not have sufficient numbers of vitamins, enzymes or even fiber to aid in the digestive process. The food you eat should provide at least some of the ingredients needed to help in its digestion, otherwise you may not even be gaining the benefits from it at all, no matter how many nutrients they contain. This is true of any processed food even if the processing is only cooking; the more a food is processed, the fewer enzymes it has. Enzymes are an important part of the digestive and nutrient assimilation process.[30]

Secondly, whole foods provide balance in the body that processed or partial foods cannot provide. For example, eggs became the great evil about fifteen years ago when they were discovered to "raise cholesterol levels", so people started avoiding them. However, eggs also contain lecithin that balance cholesterol intake in the body.[31] So as a whole food, eggs are healthy, but as an incomplete food (yolks used alone in custards), they are not.

Processed foods are also very inefficient to eat. You must eat more of them to satisfy the body so you may gain weight by eating too much food. Our bodies are satisfied nutritionally[32]- not by volume - and every organ is dependent on its nutriment from the intestinal tract so this is very important.[33] Foods like wheat grass contain super-high amounts of nutrients. One pound of wheat grass is equal in nutrient value to nearly twenty-five pounds of the choicest vegetables. A single serving of sprouts on a salad supplies half the RDA of vitamin C for an adult.[34] There are no processed foods that can make these claims honestly. This fact is made clear just by looking at the nutrient values on a package of rice cakes or granola bars. Manufacturers try to claim their products contain high nutrient value, but they can only claim that by adding synthetic vitamins and minerals to their products which are not useful to the human body. The elements of organic minerals are loosely held together so that when they enter the body they can be easily assimilated. However, the constituent parts of inorganic minerals are held together by bonds so tight that the body cannot easily break them and rarely benefits from the consumption of them. [35]

The Fourth Building Block of Health: Don't Eat Fake Food

Examples in Scriptures of the Virtues of Real Foods:
- *"Eat of the Good foods we have provided you"* (Koran 7:160)
- *"They ask thee what is lawful to them (as food). Say: Lawful unto you are (all) things good and pure."* (Koran 5:4)
- *"The mothers shall give suck to their offspring for two whole years."* (Koran 2:223)
- *"You are to distinguish between the holy and the common, and between the unclean and the clean."* (Leviticus 10:10: Old Testament[36])
- *"For the ear tests words as the palate tastes food.* (Job 34:3: Bible)
- *"Do not desire his delicacies, for they are deceptive food."* (Proverbs 23:3:Bible)
- *"For the mountains yield food for him where all the wild beasts play."* (Job 40:20:Bible)
- *"Man ate of the bread of the angels; he sent them food in abundance."* (Psalms 78:25:)
- *"Thou dost cause the grass to grow for the cattle, and plants for man to cultivate, that he may bring forth food from the earth."* (Psalms 104:14: Bible)
- *"All grain is ordained for the use of man and of beasts, to be the staff of life, not only for man but for the beasts of the field, and the fowls of heaven, and all wild animals that run or creep on the earth; And these hath God made for the use of man only in times of famine and excess of hunger. All grain is good for the food of man; as also the fruit of the vine; that which yieldeth fruit, whether in the ground or above the ground— Nevertheless, wheat for man, and corn for the ox, and oats for the horse, and rye for the fowls and for swine, and for all beasts of the field, and barley for all useful animals, and for mild drinks, as also other grain."* (Doctrine & Covenants 89:12,15-17)

15

The fourth block of health is to eat real foods and not "fake" foods. Fake foods are foods that have been tampered with on such a large scale that some of them are not even food anymore, although we often believe they are. Margarine, for example, is one of these foods. Chemically it is "one step away from being plastic"[37] Other fake foods include irradiated foods, hybrid seed produce, foods grown with pesticides, and foods with added chemicals and colors.

Foods with added chemicals and colors are the worst danger we face in our diet today. Artificial sweeteners alone can account for many of the health problems we encounter on a daily basis. These artificial sweeteners, no matter how healthy they claim to be, actually increase appetite in general and increase preference for fat intake. They also interfere with the body's ability to select foods containing the nutrients it needs. Chemicals are even worse. The list of chemicals that are added to food and what they do is thousands of pages long and growing. One example is the methyl xanthine contained in coffee, colas, teas and chocolate. It causes a common sensitivity response in some women known as fibrostic breast disease.[38] Some foods, are so "fake", in fact that our bodies reject them altogether. Numerous studies on sodium chloride show that our body excretes nearly as much as it takes in all day[39]showing that common table salt is not being used by our bodies at all.

However, not all toxic things are excreted from our body so easily. And even when they are, they may have already done some damage. Preservatives, for instance, can be classified with poisonous drugs because they have the same ill effect on the tissues in which they settle.[40]And when toxins settle in the body from food, they don't just effect the alimentary tract. All the organs depend on the blood which flows through the colon for nutrients so they absorb all the toxins present there. A person definitely needs to   develop a label-reading skill when they shop. However, even then there is no guarantee - not all the chemicals in the package have to be listed on the label. Only if a processor substitutes or adds a non-standard chemical must they report it. Ice cream, for instance has up to thirty additives that do not have to appeal on the label.[41]

Even more horrifying is that the American Medical Association's approval of food (which is the final step before it is allowed to market) simply indicates that the product is disease and bacteria free. They have no standard for what nutrient values the food must contain or even that it must even resemble at all its original source![42]

Surprisingly enough some of the supplements intended to "enrich" our whole foods and "make them whole again" are some of the worst fake foods you can find. In fact, when we take supplements, even   good ones, we are getting isolated elements that we should be getting from whole foods. Dr. Ted Morter, in his book Your Health...Your Choice says, "Its much like taking a statement out of context, you might get the full benefit of it but more likely what you get is distorted". Supplements may also cause you to feel better for some time, as they add stimulation and nutrients you need to parts of your body, but over time you will find you need more and more supplements to feel as good, and that you are becoming dependent on supplements. This is because supplements are able to add stimulation to the body in the short term, but they cannot correct the cause of your problem.[43] Supplements, for this reason should never be taken in isolation over a long period of time, but should only be used to correct chronic health problems in the short term. The long term solution for your health must come from real and whole foods. The only acceptable long-term supplements are those made from whole foods such as dried barley, wheat grass, vegetables, fruits or greens. However, even these can cause an imbalance in the body over time if they are taken daily as they do not provide the wide spectrum or variety of nutrients the body needs over a long period of time.

Another interesting fact about fake foods is that they often cause allergic reactions in people when the "real" version of the food does not. In fact, produce contaminated by antibiotics, bacteria and hormones cause problems for people who, when eating the same organic produce, are fine.[44] Furthermore, organic produce has a higher nutrient content than produce grown with all these pesticides.[45] An average of two hundred pounds of chemical fertilizer is used per acre every year on non-organic crops.[46]

Perhaps our mass consumption of all these fake foods is what prompted Abram Hoffer, MD, Ph.D. and Walter Morton, DPM, to say, "The American junk diet is the Western form of malnutrition."[47]

The Fifth Building Block of Health: Eat Raw Foods

Examples in Scriptures of the Virtues of Raw Foods:

- *"And God said, "Behold, I have given you every plant yielding seed which is upon the face of all the earth, and every tree with seed in its fruit; you shall have them for food"* (Genesis 1:29: Bible)
- *"Then to eat of all the produce of the earth and find with skill the spacious Paths of the Lord; there issues from within their bodies a drink of varying colors wherein is healing for men."* (16:69: Koran)
- *Every herb in the season thereof, and every fruit in the season thereof; all these to be used with prudence and thanksgiving.* (Doctrine & Covenants 89:11)

The fifth building block of health is to eat raw foods. In fact, humans are the *only species* on earth that try to exist on cooked enzymeless meals without the proper balance of raw and living foods![48] Enzymes are the catalyst that help substances to either combine or break down in our body. They are important in every bodily function and cooked foods do not have them. The body *does* produce a limited amount of its own enzymes and also stores enzymes. Despite this fact, we need these enzymes for use in repairing and rebuilding our body in times of illness or stress.[49] If we use all of our body's stored enzymes up just to help us digest our food (which we eat too much of anyway!) then we won't have them when we are sick and really need them.

When raw plants are eaten the enzymes contained in the plants assist our digestive system to process the food we just ate. Without enzymes the food we eat is "dead" so raw food is sometimes referred to as "living" food. That does not mean we should be eating live cows, however, to get our meat. Cooking changes the nature of the bonds that hold food together and makes them stronger and less digestible but cooking also has some benefits and recent research has shown that cooking, although it also destroys some nutrients, also enhances or reveals others.[50] So most natural health advocates recommend starting out by eating at least 30% raw foods and then moving up to 75% raw if you can manage.[51] But how raw does raw food have to be? Even low to moderate heat (118 degrees) destroys most enzymes.[52] In fact, most of what we *do* to food destroys enzymes and nutrients in our food .Peeling, boiling, cooking, roasting, baking and poaching all destroy minerals in our food.[53]

So should we eat meat raw? Most people cannot handle raw meat. However milk is an animal product one should try to obtain raw. Milk appears to be a raw food (it just comes straight out of the cow doesn't it?) but it is not. Once milk is pasteurized the bonds that hold the minerals together are altered and the calcium may not be as usable. Even calves die on pasteurized milk.[54]

The Sixth Building Block of Health: Eat Foods Appropriately

Examples in Scriptures of the Virtues of Appropriate Eating:

- *"These all look to thee, to give them their food in due season."* (Psalms 104:27:Bible)
- *"Eat of the good things We have provided for your sustenance but commit no excess therein"* (Koran 20:81)
- *"If you will diligently hearken to the voice of the Lord your God, and do that which is right in His eyes, and give heed to His commandments and keep all His statutes, I will put none of the diseases upon you which I put upon the Egyptians; for I am the Lord, your healer."* (Exodus15:26: Bible)
- *"Take care of yourself, and guard your soul diligently"* (Deuteronomy 4:9: Old Testament)
- *"Yea, flesh also of beasts and of the fowls of the air, I, the Lord, have ordained for the use of man with thanksgiving; nevertheless they are to be used sparingly; And it is pleasing unto me that they should not be used, only in times of winter, or of cold, or famine."* (Doctrine & Covenants 89:13,14)

The sixth building block of health is to eat foods appropriately. Eating foods appropriately means that foods should be eaten by who they were meant to be eaten by, how they were meant to be eaten, when they were meant to be eaten, and in combinations that are suitable. As a nation we are eating any food we want at any time and combining it in any way we want without any thought to the benefit or harm we are doing to our bodies. Even worse, with the emergence of international trading and the ease of shopping in mega grocery stores we are able to get foods from all corners of the earth even if we have lived in the same town our entire lives.

Eating the food *you* were meant to be eating refers to eating foods that belong in your type or category. Abram Hoffer, MD, in his book, Putting it all Together: The New Ortomolecular Nutrition, says, *"The range of variation between individuals is enormous. Some people become violently ill from ingesting foods that are nutritious for others. This truth explodes the myth of the RDAs.* "[55]

All systems of natural medicine have some sort of category of types to use as a guideline. There is not any evidence that one system is better than another, but there is evidence that using A system is better than using NO system. The Chinese system of healing divides people into dry, damp, hot, cold, deficient and excess.[56] The Ayurvedic system divides people into vata, pitta & kapha (air water and fire)[57]. In the Ayurvedic system the Vata (air) predominant type is prone to neurological disorders, coldness, and dryness. Foods that have cool energy, dry and rough qualities with bitter or astringent tastes aggravate Vata. Vata should instead have warm, moist, nourishing, sweet and salty and sour foods.[58]Bernard Jensen's system based on Rocine's system of types divides people into categories corresponding to the various minerals such as calcium, magnesium and sulphur.[59] In his guidelines he mentions that people who are mentally high strung should eat more calcium foods since it is one of the greatest elements used to "ground" people. People who use their brains a great deal use up phosphorus and need to increase their intake of that mineral.[60] Many years of experimentation and observation led Rocine to the understanding that different people, due to inherent temperament metabolic disposition, mental activity and predominant faculties use the basic chemical elements at different rates, producing chemicals in the body which then correspond to distinct types. He identified 20 types of people.[61]One bestseller in 1997, called Eat Right for your Type divides people into four blood groups.

Eating right for a condition or type takes a lot of planning. One needs to be aware of what foods are not suitable for them, which foods *are* suitable and what various foods will do in general. Many people may have figured this out for themselves by the time they learned new system of eating. If a person is not able to follow an exact system of eating for their type they should at least be aware of what various foods do to different people and what foods they are allergic or sensitive to. This awareness will enable them to "eat for their type" at least on a moderate level.

For instance, contractive foods like meat and salt cause the body to draw in or contract it resources inward (to help in the digestion of these complex foods). The body must devote a lot of resources to processing contractive foods. This energy will eventually rebound out in the form of a temper tantrum or some other outburst. Expansive foods like fruits, on the other hand, cause the body to expand outwards and keep energy levels on the surface. So when a person eats a lot of fruit their energy tends to stay on the surface and is expressed intensely. They may seem "up in the clouds" a lot. Obviously someone with a temper should avoid eating a lot of meat and someone with a problem concentrating should avoid eating too much fruit.[62] Bernard Jensen emphasizes this when says, "We need to be very cautious of the vibratory rate of meat which is very stimulating to the ego centers of the brain which can be very destructive." Although he also states that, "Nearly all of the oldest people I encountered in my travels around the world were meat eaters."[63] so apparently meat is not a forbidden factor in health and longevity either.

Eating foods one is allergic to, should also be avoided. In fact, being allergic to foods could be an indicator of what food type a person is. By avoiding foods one has a sensitivity or aversion to they may be naturally eating for their type. This is one reason children should not be forced to eat things they dislike. As long as they are offered a variety of healthy, whole, and raw foods at each meal, the child should be able to chose which he or she likes from this selection. Take note that being allergic to a food does not mean that one will break out in hives or have an asthma attack. A person may notice more subtle reactions such as headaches, itching in the throat, indigestion, or perhaps even just an unexplainable aversion to the food. Sometimes a person may even experience the opposite - an extreme obsession with the food. However small or large the reaction is, though, do not brush it aside. Jacqueline Krohn, in her book The Whole Way to Allergy Relief and Prevention warns, *"If you continue to eat foods to which you're allergic, without rotation or extracts you will experience reactions with every meal and snack. Continued reactions over a long period of time will weaken your immune system."*[64]

Eating right for a type may also include taking into account age, weight, sex or nationality. Women, for instance, lose calcium through menstruation and need to be aware of that fact once a month in their diet plan.[65] The elderly need to be more careful about food combining in general because their systems are weaker and less able to tolerate excesses in diet. In children the thyroid does not begin to function until they are two to five years old so they should be supplied with extra iodine rich foods to protect them from toxins.[66]

Nonetheless, and despite all the rules and regulations of these systems, the wisest, easiest and most natural way to "eat right for a type" is to simply eat what is around and what is in season. Donald Lepore, an expert on Kinesiology and allergy prevention believes, "God did not permit foods that are antagonistic to man's existence to be grown in the area of consumption".[67] I agree with him. We can often avoid most of our problems by simply eating foods that are grown nearby and in season, and perhaps adding or subtracting from this selection according to our age, stage (pregnant, nursing, man or woman), and tastes (we should still avoid items we are allergic to). This is perhaps one of the best arguments for shopping at the farmer's market instead of the grocery store. At the farmer's market consumers can buy what is fresh, grows around them and is in season. At the grocery store shoppers will find fruits and vegetables from all over the world, and usually picked before they are ripe so as to lengthen their shelf life. Immature fruits and vegetables are deficient in sodium content among other things.[68] We also need to be aware of the season for non-produce items when we are shopping. Barley heats the blood and thus makes a wonderful winter soup but is not very advisable in the hot summer months.[69]

The order and combination of foods is also very important in how they affect the health. Deciding which foods to combine in which order may seem difficult, but there are actually only a few basic rules to follow. The first rule is that fresh fruit must not be eaten with any other food, even dried fruit. Fruit is classified as a pre-digested food which moves straight through the stomach and into the intestines. When it combines with any other food in the stomach it will ferment itself and anything else in the stomach.[70] This is perhaps the easiest rule to remember because traditionally fresh fruit is always eaten alone as a snack or desert item (Without whip cream or cobbler crust). However, the easiest way to remember proper food combination is to know *why* certain combinations work and why others do not work. When a person understands why some combinations don't work, then they will not have trouble remembering the rules.

The second rule of food combining is to start each meal off with something raw.[71] The reason is because raw foods contain the enzymes that help us to digest our food. Furthermore, just like the first rule, this is also a traditional practice in most cultures. Traditionally and formally the salads and hors devours (that often contain other raw items) are eaten before a meal. So the answer to, "Why do we eat salads first and deserts last?" lies in the laws of proper food order and combining.

The third rule of food combining is to not mix protein and starches. One may eat starches with vegetables and vegetables with meat, but should try to avoid combining starches and proteins.[72] The reason is that proteins and starches require completely different environments for digestion. If a person combines them, neither will end up having the ideal environment. This will not make a person sick, but will simply mean that what they are eating is not being digested and utilized to the most of its ability which means they are not getting the benefit from the food they are eating which means they will need to eat more food and to have more nutrients as well. Proteins need a more acidic environment for digestion while carbohydrates and starches can be prepared for digestion at a much quicker rate.[73] Furthermore, a protein meal takes up to five hours to be digested so it should be the last meal of the day since your body needs to concentrate on digesting it.

"How much" is also a factor when considering what to eat. Moderation is always a good choice. If all the foods you choose are whole and natural it would be hard to find something wrong with eating them. But anything in excess can be detrimental to your health and this is clearly illustrated in our consumption of two substances: proteins and sugar. Abram Hoffer, MD, author of Putting it all Together: The New Orthomolecular Nutrition states that, *"The only difference between sugar addiction and heroin addiction is that sugar does not need an injection."*[74] and Dr. Ted Morter, author of YourHealth...YourChoice states that "Too much protein leads to toxicity"[75]

Excess protein consumption leads to an over acid environment in the body. This environment does not allow the normal cellular functions of the body to perform correctly and causes leaching of minerals from the organs. In fact, as little as forty seven grams of protein a day can cause your body to lose more calcium than you take in with your food.[76] It is difficult to see protein as a culprit, though, since a plump fried chicken can taste so good and keep one full for so long. It seems that something that tastes good and gives us so much energy cannot be "bad". However, the fact that we are full for so long is not necessarily good news for our digestive system. It may be annoying to feel hungry every two or three hours, but it is even more annoying to the body to have the heavy protein load of meat sitting in the intestines for five hours or more. The more a food sits in the body, the more chance the body has of soaking up toxins from that substance and if one eats non- organic meats, their body is soaking up even more than toxins. It is soaking up hormones and antibiotics as well. In fact, the higher people eat up the food chain, from grains to fruits to leafy vegetables and all the way up to milk, eggs and animal meats, the higher the concentration of pesticides and other chemical pollutants are in the food. Dairy products alone have a 250% increase in toxins over leafy vegetables and a 1500% increase over root vegetables.

Another deceptive thing about protein is that it gives us so much energy. We usually eat food to give us energy so this seems like a good thing. However, protein does not increase energy - it stimulates *nervous* energy. In fact protein is second only to drugs as a major stimulant. Even coffee, cola drinks and tea are weak stimulants compared to protein.[77]

Sugar is another deceptive food. Sugar tastes good and enhances the taste of many other substances. However, sugar increases appetite, interferes with digestion of foods, and leaches vitamins and minerals out of the system (especially calcium and sodium). Basically, sugar harms us by stimulating the physiological activity of the body into action, but then not providing any enzymes, vitamins or minerals to process it. So it then must take the nutrients it needs from the body to process itself in the body. This leaves us with a shortage of nutrients which causes us to feel hungrier and in the long run may cause visible nutrient deficiencies.[78] Many people, believing that only white sugar is bad, use honey or other sweeteners as a substitute, but *all* sugars and sweeteners (even honey) ultimately have similar effects on the body even if some substances show these effects stronger than others.

Nancy Appleton, MD, who wrote Lick the Sugar Habit lists the following things that sugar can do to our body: Suppress the immune system (three soft drinks will wipe out the immune system for the day); upset the minerals in the body; cause hyperactivity, anxiety, and difficulty concentrating; produce a significant rise in triglycerides, cause reduction in defense against bacterial infection, cause kidney damage, reduce high density lipoproteins, lead to chromium deficiency, lead to breast, ovarian or prostate cancer; increase fasting levels of glucose and insulin, cause copper deficiency, interfere with absorption of calcium and magnesium, weaken eyesight, raise the levels of neurotransmitters called seratonin, cause hypoglycemia, produce acidic stomach, cause aging, arthritis, asthma, candida, gallstones, appendicitis, heart disease, varicose veins, and periodontal disease; increase cholesterol and migraine headaches; interfere with the absorption of protein, cause toxemia during pregnancy, impair the structure of DNA, cause cataracts; and cause hunger pangs and overeating.

Artificial sweeteners are even more dangerous. Aspartame, long considered a "safe" sugar substitute and the one people turn to to try to avoid all the sugar problems listed above actually may cause more problems than the sugar people are trying to avoid. This is not surprising considering that Aspartame breaks all the rules of a healthy food. It is not raw, it is not whole, and it is a fake food. Aspartame is made of phenylalanine, aspartic acid (two amino acids) and methanol (commonly known as methyl alcohol or wood alcohol). Consumption of Aspartame can cause a flooding of amino acids in the bloodstream, blindness, brain swelling, and inflammation of the pancreas and heart. Aspartame has also been reported to cause headaches, mood swings, changes in vision, nausea and diarrhea, sleep disorders, memory loss and confusion and convulsions. It is especially unsafe for children.[79]

The Seventh Building Block of Health: Exercise

Examples in Scriptures of the Virtues of Exercise:

- *"When My servants ask thee concerning Me, I am indeed close (to them): I respond to the prayer of every suppliant when he calleth on Me: Let them also, with a will, Listen to My call, and believe in Me: That they may walk in the right way."* (Koran 2:186)[80]

The physical bending, prostating act of prayer, performed five times a day by all Muslims is said by some to have physical benefits of those similar to exercise. [81]

- *"Arise, walk through the length and the breadth of the land, for I will give it to you."* (Genesis 13:17: Old Testament)
- *"After this he appeared in another form to two of them, as they were walking into the country."* (Mark 16:12:Bible)
- *"And they were on the road, going up to Jerusalem, and Jesus was walking ahead of them; and they were amazed, and those who followed were afraid. And taking the twelve again, he began to tell them what was to happen to him."* (Mark 10:32)
- *"And shall run and not be weary, and shall walk and not faint."* (Doctrine & Covenants 89:20)

The seventh building block of health is exercise. Exercise is the motion that causes the body to circulate the good nutrients we (hopefully) put into it. Bernard Jensen says that *"A body can become anemic with the best blood stream in the world if the blood does not circulate fast enough."*[82] Exercise is what gets the blood moving and keeps it moving. A healthy flow of blood means better assimilation, less time for toxins to settle and quicker elimination. A good indication for how important exercise is to bodily function is that after surgery, when a person must be confined to bed, it is found that muscles, nerves, and many body functions begin to suffer from just a few days of inactivity.[83]

Exercise does not have to be formal or vigorous for it to be beneficial. Walking in the grass before breakfast helps stimulate blood to circulate in the extremities and barefoot *walking* (not jogging) is the best method of developing the small muscles which help return blood to the heart.[84] In fact, a brisk walk can so efficiently get the blood flowing and body clearing itself that a walk can even clear allergic reactions.[85]

Exercise is an extremely important part of any health maintenance program. As Ted Morter says in his book, Your Health...Your Choice, *"Health is served at the meal table, muscles and stamina are built by exercise."*[86] However, Morter calls exercise *"the cherry on top"* meaning that exercise is an addition to good eating and not a substitute for it. You cannot get healthy by exercising or having a personal trainer at the gym. You must first eat healthy so when you exercise your body has the right fuel to pump through it. In fact, too much exercise combined with the wrong eating habits can even be deadly. For instance, if a person has a large meal with an acidifying effect on the body (as most of our American meals are) and the goes out to exercise, this person can die from the over acidity in their body. Exercise itself causes the acidity level in the blood to rise and acid on top of acid in the body can be fatal.[87] Perhaps this is part of the wisdom behind the often-disputed rule, "Don't go swimming on a full stomach."

Exercise is even more important in cases of recovery. Anne Frahm, in her book A Cancer Battle Plan, lists three reasons that exercise is beneficial for recovery: to provide emotional nourishment, to alleviate family fears, to relieve fears and tension, and to strengthen the recovering body as it stimulates the immune system. She says that exercise is emotionally nourishing because when patients realize they can be active and do normal activities like go to the gym, they become less fearful. The families themselves also become less fearful for the patient, and tend to see them more as a "person recovering" than a "person with cancer".[88]

The Eighth Building Block of Health: Use Pure Water & Breathe Fresh Air

Examples in Scriptures of the Virtues of Pure Air and Water:[89]

- *"And when he had said this, he <u>breathed</u> on them, and said to them, "Receive the Holy Spirit."* (John 20:22: Bible)
- *"But man dies, and is laid low; man <u>breathes</u> his last, and where is he?"* (Job 14:10)
- *"Let everything that <u>breathes</u> praise the LORD! Praise the LORD!"* (Psalms 105:6: Bible)
- *"And they said, An Egyptian delivered us out of the hand of the shepherds, and also drew [water] abundantly for us, and <u>watered</u> the flock."* (Exodus 2:19: Old Testament)
- *"When they came to Marah, they could not drink the <u>water</u> of Marah because it was bitter; therefore it was named Marah."* (Exodus 15:23: Old Testament)
- *"And he cried to the LORD; and the LORD showed him a tree, and he threw it into the <u>water</u>, and the <u>water</u> became sweet. There the LORD made for them a statute and an*

ordinance and there he proved them." (Exodus 15:25: Bible)

- *"Then they came to Elim, where there were twelve springs of <u>water</u> and seventy palm trees; and they encamped there by the <u>water</u>."* (Exodus 15:27: Old Testament)
- *"And remember Moses prayed for <u>water</u> for his people; We said: "Strike the rock with thy staff." Then gushed forth therefrom twelve springs. Each group knew its own place for <u>water</u>. So eat and drink of the sustenance provided by Allah, and do no evil nor mischief on the (face of the) earth."* (Koran 2:60)
- *"In front of such a one is Hell, and he is given, for drink, boiling fetid <u>water</u>."* (Koran 14:16)
- *"The righteous (will be) amid Gardens and fountains (of clear-flowing <u>water</u>)."* (Koran 15:45)
- *"Narrated Abu Huraira: Allah's Apostle said, "If a fly falls in the vessel of any of you, let him dip all of it (into the vessel) and then throw it away, for in one of its wings there is a disease and in the other there is healing (antidote for it) i e. the treatment for that disease."* (Muslim Sahih Buhkari: Volume 7, Book 71, Number 673)
- *"We made <u>water</u> essential for every life"* (Koran 21:30)
- *"The human being has never filled a container worse than his stomach. Hense it would be sufficient for the son of Adam to satisfy his hunger with a few bites to strengthen his backbone. If he must eat his fill then he should allow for one third food, one third <u>water</u> and one third <u>air</u>."* (Hadith of the Prophet Muhammad: Masnad)
- *"You shall serve the Lord your God, and I will bless your bread and your <u>water</u>; and I will take sickness away from the midst of you. None shall cast her young or be barren in your land; I will fulfill the number of your days".* (Exodus 23:25,26 Old Testament)
- *"Yea, and ye also know that Moses, by his word according to the power of God which was in him, smote the rock, and there came forth <u>water</u>, that the children of Israel might quench their thirst. "* (Book of Mormon 1 Nephi 17:29)

The eighth principal of health is to drink pure water and breathe fresh air. As a nation we are obsessed with what we eat and what supplements we can take, but we often overlook the two most obvious sources of our health problems - water and air. The human body is two thirds water and this water is involved in every bodily process including digestion, absorption, circulation and excretion.[90] We take in from 300-400 gallons of air per day to keep us alive[91] and the one thing we cannot last without for even a few minutes is air. We can go without water for a few days and food for perhaps a month. But without air we die very quickly. It is amazing, then, with the importance of these two substances that we worry much about our food at all!

The six ways we can absorb toxins from our water is to drink it, cook with it, buy canned products canned with it, swim in it, bathe in it, or shower in it. If a person is drinking, cooking with and showering with water from the tap and swimming in the local pool they are absorbing toxins. All water that comes into public systems has its source in contamination. In the original water source there may be parasites, virus, herbicides, pesticides, cyanides, asbestos, and industrial chemicals. Even residues from pesticides used decades ago may still be present in the water system today.[92] This polluted water is then treated with chlorine, fluoride, carbon, lime, phosphates, soda, ash, and aluminum sulfate to "purify" it, then sent through zinc and cadmium pipe joints and copper pipes to our home. It is ironic that we use chemicals to combat the chemicals and pollutants that are already in the water. It is like adding insult to injury. To be precise, forty seven "insults" in all are added to our water to disinfect, fluoridate, soften, coagulate, chlorinate, oxidate, condition, neutralize, and control odor and color.[93] Among these chemicals are chlorine and fluoride. Chlorine can cause allergic reactions and can either be absorbed or ingested and leaches potassium and sodium from the body, causing an electrolyte depletion.[94] The salts used to fluoridate our nation's water supply, sodium fluoride and florosamicic acid are industrial byproducts that are never found in nature. They are so toxic they are used in rat poisons as well.[95] We can get all the natural fluorine we need from fish, bones, quince and raw goats milk.[96]

Unfortunately, the only way to remove fluorine from your water is to use reverse osmosis, distillation or activated aluminum filtration. All of these systems are very expensive and they all have drawbacks as well, the main drawback being that the water is being processed to such a great extent that in the end you are drinking just H20 and not just plain pure natural water anymore. Distilled water can even be detrimental to the health if used over the long term as it leaches minerals from the body when we drink it. Many people think the worst thing about distilled water is that its nutrient value has been eliminated, but do not realize that it also *leaches* minerals from the body. Long-term use affects the mineral storage facilities in the body.[97] Nevertheless, experts agree that a water lacking in its original nutrients is still superior to water laden with chemicals and toxins, so to use the best water you can, you need to filter it in some way. All filters remove dirt, rust and sediment, although some do a better job than others. Most department store filters will take out 98% of chlorine, and up to 95% of heavy metals such as lead, aluminum, mercury and copper, significantly reducing zinc, cadmium, and sulfates. More sophisticated filters like the Katadyn will take out 100% of parasites, cysts and bacteria. In between there are many choices. You can get a countertop distiller, a six-step ultraviolet sterilization unit, and reverse osmosis units with varying degrees of advancement. In the end you need to choose the system that suits you. A system that claims 100% removal of bacteria would be overkill for someone who has water coming from a city system that has already killed all the bacteria with the chlorine. A person living in a farming district would want to make sure they have a unit that filters pesticides, and a person in the suburbs or city may want to get their water tested before they make a final decision on what they will use. A person can also buy water in bottles but they need to be careful as, much of the "bottled water" today is just as good as what comes out of the tap *without* a filter.

Air is the other major substance we need to purify around our homes. Air is so valuable, in fact, that people in polluted areas such as Los Angeles have only one thousandth as much air to breathe as they would under normal conditions. [98] A professor or Entomology and Agricultural science has reported that 65% of the pesticides used in the USA are applied by aircraft and that about 50-75% of this ends up in the environment while only 25% hits the intended target.[99] Cleaning and personal care products are other big air pollution offenders. Formaldehyde, found in air fresheners, glue and moth balls can cause breathing problems in many people.[100] Many more people are allergic or sensitive to synthetic scents and other chemicals found in cleaners, air fresheners, aroma candles, deodorants, dish soap, laundry soap, perfumes, deodorant sprays, shampoos and more. By not using natural products in our bathrooms and cleaning buckets we are just adding more pollution to our air. Some pollutants can be removed with sophisticated air filters and some houseplants such as the spider plant, are very good air filters. However, the best way to avoid air pollution is to try to live in a place far from traffic, factories or other industrial pollutants, to use natural cleaning products and to use natural personal care products.

The Ninth Building Block of Health: Hygiene

Examples in Scriptures of the Virtues of Hygiene:
- *"...and He loves those who keep themselves pure and <u>clean</u>."* (Koran 2:222)
- *"Or if any one touches an un<u>clean</u> thing, whether the carcass of an un<u>clean</u> beast or a carcass of un<u>clean</u> cattle or a carcass of un<u>clean</u> swarming things, and it is hidden from him, and he has become un<u>clean</u>, he shall be guilty."* (Leviticus 5:2: Old Testament)
- *"And when he who has a discharge is cleansed of his discharge, then he shall count for himself seven days for his cleansing, and wash his clothes; and he shall bathe his body in running water, and shall be clean."* (Leviticus 5:13: Old Testament)
- *"Jesus said to him, "He who has <u>bathed</u> does not need to wash, except for his feet, but he is <u>clean</u> all over; and you are <u>clean</u>, but not every one of you."* (John 13:10: New Testament)
- *"Approach not prayers with mind befogged...and until after washing your whole body..."* (4:43: Koran)
- *"But thou, when thou fastest, anoint thy head, and wash thy face"* (Book of Mormon 3 Nephi 13:17)
- *"And, again, strong drinks are not for the belly, but for the washing of your bodies."* (Doctrine & Covenants 89:7)

The ninth principal of health is to keep good hygiene. The skin is the largest organ on the body and performs much of the elimination job of toxins from the body. When this organ is clogged with dirt or sweat that has not been washed off, it cannot perform its job properly. Water, mild soap and perhaps a luffa sponge are sufficient for this purpose although some people consider a luffa essential as it buffs the old skin cells from the skin, allowing the new ones to flourish, and the old ones to avoid clogging. Brushing of the teeth is also very important. New evidence has linked everything from cancer to heart disease back to periodontal disease. The theory is that germs and bacteria can enter the blood stream through unhealthy pockets in the teeth and cause disease. Prevention is emphasized in this category.

The Tenth Building Block of Health: Use Nature to Heal
Examples in Scriptures of the Using Nature to Heal:

- *"God never inflicts a disease unless he makes a cure for it..."* (Hadith of the Prophet Muhammad related by Abu Hurairah)
- *" And when I sicken, God heals me"* (26:80 Koran)
- *"And whosoever among you are sick , and have not faith to be healed, but believe, shall be nourished with all tenderness, with herbs and mild food"* (Doctrine & Covenants 42:43)

The prophet of Islam, Muhammad, was known for his skill as a natural and spiritual healer, using various natural therapies, herbs, foods and even recitations of the Koran to heal people. His knowledge and guidance have been written down in at least 30 volumes of his life practices, as well as hundreds of books on Prophetic Medicine, a handful of which have been translated into English.

- *"Through the middle of the street of the city; also, on either side of the river, the tree of life with its twelve kinds of fruit, yielding its fruit each month; and the leaves of the tree were for the healing of the nations."* (Revelations: Bible)
- *"Go up to Gilead, and take balm, O virgin daughter of Egypt! In vain you have used many medicines; there is no healing for you."* (Jeremiah 46:11: Bible)
- *"And on the banks, on both sides of the river, there will grow all kinds of trees for food. Their leaves will not wither nor their fruit fail, but they will bear fresh fruit every month, because the water for them flows from the sanctuary. Their fruit will be for food, and their leaves for healing."* (Ezekiel 47:12: Old Testament)
- *Narrated Abu Said Al-Khudri: A man came to the Prophet and said, "My brother has some abdominal trouble." The Prophet said to him "Let him drink honey." The man came for the second time and the Prophet said to him, 'Let him drink honey." He came for the third time and the Prophet said, "Let him drink honey." He returned again and said, "I have done that ' The Prophet then said, "Allah has said the truth, but your brother's abdomen has told a lie. Let him drink honey." So he made him drink honey and he was cured.* (Volume 7, Book 71, Number 588: Sahih Bukhari: Muslim)
- *"Narrated Um Qais bint Mihsan: I heard the Prophet saying, "Treat with the Indian incense, for it has healing for seven diseases; it is to be sniffed by one having throat trouble, and to be put into one side of the mouth of one suffering from pleurisy." Once I went to Allah's Apostle with a son of mine who would not eat any food, and the boy passed urine on him whereupon he asked for some water and sprinkled it over the place of urine."* (Volume 7, Book 71, Number 596: Sahih Bukhari: Muslim)
- *Narrated 'Aisha: The Prophet used to treat some of his wives by passing his right hand over the place of ailment and used to say, "O Allah, the Lord of the people! Remove the*

trouble and heal the patient, for You are the Healer. No healing is of any avail but Yours; healing that will leave behind no ailment." (Volume 7, Book 71, Number 639: Sahih Bukhari: Muslim)

- *"Narrated Said bin Zaid: I heard the Prophet saying, "Truffles are like Manna (i.e. they grow naturally without man's care) and their water heals eye diseases."* (Volume 7, Book 71, Number 609: Sahih Bukhari: Muslim)

The tenth principal of health is to use natural therapies and substances to heal. Dr. Cheyene, MD, says, "Medical medicines are so destructive to human bodies that malice could not invent anything more deadly beyond gunpowder itself."[101] Prescription medicines mask symptoms, cause damage to our bodies, contain harmful chemicals, are often fatal in certain combinations, and are often prescribed without proper knowledge or testing. Finally, after all that trouble, they do not even cure.

Yet, even though there are numerous studies to prove that prescription medicines are dangerous and natural medicines are safe, people still hold onto the idea that herbs can't heal them as well as the chemicals can. Why is this? Perhaps because of the mass marketing that drug companies do lately, people are being brainwashed into believing the power of prescription medicines. It is certainly not hard to be brainwashed. In one evening of television the audience will see a full scale model of how the stomach's acid is disintegrated by a leading antacid, and another person's heartwarming tale of how a leading headache medicine gave them their life back. The pictures are so amazing, the claims so promising and the people so convincing viewers forget they are looking at actors getting paid by people who have a lot of money because they are selling this product. When the public see these pictures night after night and then read the ads again in their favorite magazine and see posters on the wall of the doctor's office, what can they do?

Yet, if pharmaceuticals are so extraordinary then why do the royal family of Great Britain steer clear of them and use only homeopathy? And why have they been using it since 1755 and enjoying a history of fantastic family health that is envied worldwide?[102] And if pharmaceuticals are so wonderful then why did Rome banish theirs after seeing the wonders of healing accomplished by Hippocrates with only a few herbs? Rome had relied on her physicians for six centuries, much longer than we have relied on ours, yet they were wise enough to see the miracle in herbal healing and were able to recover as a nation.[103] Perhaps it is time for us to "recover as a nation as well". In 1900 a health survey was taken of 110 nations and in this survey the United States ranked 13th from the top for good health. Recently another survey was taken of 79 nations and the United States ranked 79th.[104] Perhaps that is because over seventy-five percent of the world's population already use natural medicines/herbs to heal.[105] Obviously, even with all of our modern tools and medicines something is wrong.

Pharmaceuticals are not only *not* effective in the long run, but harm patients as well. Pharmaceuticals are designed to give relief to symptoms and that they do well, even if temporarily. However, they are not designed to, nor will they cure. Have you ever seen or heard an advertisement claim that their product could cure you? Of course not. And don't we all want to be cured, not just pacified? Drugs are to adults what a pacifier is to a baby - not a solution to the problem.[106] The respected herbalist Edward E. Shook said, "Disease is not cured by adding poisons to the body but by eliminating them and observing the laws of nature and aiding and assisting her in every way possible."[107] Chemical products will never cure and in the process of helping the they will just mask the symptoms meant to be a road map to the cure. When that road map is gone it is hard to tell if a patient is still sick or not, and even harder to cure them when there are no symptoms. Many people become dependent on their drugs only to die years later of suppressed symptoms of a disease they could have cured through a natural lifestyle.

Two popular over-the-counter medications are also two of the most harmful substances we put in our body: diuretics and antacids. Diuretics not only take fluid out of the body, but also the sodium, potassium, and other minerals that might be in the solution, therefore starving the body of essential nutrients.[108] Antacids ignore the fact that *most* people's problem is not too much acid in the stomach but *not enough* acid in the stomach. Health care professional Ted Morter, MA, says, "My clinical experience shows that a deficiency of gastric acid is the cause of acid indigestion" and Maesimund B. Panos, MD, author of Homeopathic Medicine at Home says, *"acid is not the villain, it is necessary for digestion..."*[109] When a person takes an antacid on a stomach with deficient hydrochloric acid, they are dissolving the little they do have. This might relieve gas pain, but the person will not assimilate any nourishment from the food they just ate.[110] Yet, this is not the least of what damage drugs can do to our bodies. They can shut down functioning organs as well. The pancreas, for example, when given insulin artificially over time will gradually lose its ability to produce the secretion of pancereatin which is absolutely necessary for the metabolism of starches.[111]

Even more horrifying is what is actually in our pharmaceuticals. Experiments show that coal tar products produce cancer in rats and guinea pigs (but who cares about the study, who would want to eat coal tar anyway?) yet about 90% of cough syrups and most of the cold remedies on the market are made from this substance.[112]

However, what is *in* our medicines is not the least of our worries. Even if the medicines themselves don't eventually kill us, certain combinations may. To date, hundreds of books are written with hundreds of pages each listing common and deadly drug-drug and drug-food combinations. Often times patients are not given this information or the doctor is not even aware of it himself. In Deadly Drug Interactions: The People's Pharmacy Guide, instead of giving case studies and statistics to prove adverse reactions the authors list under each "deadly" heading a number of *actual cases*. The sad fact is that most deadly reactions have been discovered by the patients themselves, and not in the lab before the drugs go to market.[113] This is probably why the world health organization concluded recently that one in every four people who die in hospitals is killed by prescription drugs.[114]

Even more shocking is that most of these drugs are prescribed incorrectly, either because the initial diagnosis was incorrect or because of lack of knowledge on the part of the doctor. Senator Edward Kennedy claimed, "physicians are inadequately educated about drugs in medical school, then become confused about the use of the 20,000 brand names for the 700 drug entities, and being too busy tend to rely excessively on manufacturers for drug information."[115] In fact 70% of the drugs now in use today were not even being prescribed when half of today's doctors were in medical school![116]

Misdiagnosis, however, is the biggest problem of all. Dr. Cabot stated that 50% of diagnosis made at Massachusetts General Hospital were wrong as shown by post postmortem examination. Professor Drummond, president of the British Medical association found that diagnosis was incorrect in 80% of cases shown by mortem exam.[117] Four other hospitals in this study showed similar findings.[118] If this study is any indication of the accuracy of medical diagnostics then it is easy to see how someone could get a prescription that may worsen their condition and potentially kill them.

So if all this is true then why do we persist? Why don't we frown and turn up our noses in disgust at the entire pharmaceutical industry? Perhaps because our great great great great grandmothers & grandfathers took their families to doctors that used earthworms, human excrement, hogs' lice, toads, hen skins, dried human flesh, sheep excrement to heal. Putting their trust in the medical profession of the time (instead of listening to that little voice in their head that screamed "YUUUUUCK!") they consumed the "drugs" they were given happily and without argument.[119] I believe that in the future our great great great grandchildren will look back on our medicines with the same disgust we feel now thinking about digesting sheep excrement and hogs' lice. So how are herbs better? Herbs do not have any of the "side effects" listed above. They do not mask symptoms, cause damage to our bodies, or contain harmful chemicals. They are rarely fatal when used wisely, and never fatal when combined with foods like drugs can be, and even if they are prescribed without proper knowledge or testing they do not cause the swift damage prescription drugs do. Finally, they *do* have the ability to cure you.

Herbs do not mask symptoms, they work with the body to heal rather than against it. If a person has a fever, a homeopathic or herbal remedy will bring the fever down below the danger level but it will not eliminate the fever altogether as the fever is a needed part of the cure.

Herbs also do not do damage to our bodies or contain harmful chemicals. Even herbs with strong chemical components have other components that help balance the stronger ones. Herbalists contend that nature provides the ingredients in herbs to balance the more powerful ingredients and that the pharmaceutical industry that was originally based on isolating ingredients in herbs, does not maintain this balance.[120]

Herbs will also rarely harm people when taken wisely. As long as humans avoid the toxic herbs the rest of the herbs are rarely fatal or even harmful when taken incorrectly or in large doses. In fact, nature has a built in alarm system for most herbs. If you ingest too much of an herb a person will most likely get sick before they get gravely ill or die. Nature gives us a warning that something is wrong. Most pharmaceuticals don't ring any alarm bells before they kill. Even more amazing is that some herbs appear to work only when needed. Ginseng, for instance, appears to have little effect in the absence of stress, but when stress occurs, it encourages a faster response of the stress hormones.[121]

Some herbal cures are even foods themselves and completely harmless. Blackberry vinegar, an exotic food item, is good for fevers. Ginger, a common spice warms the body in the winter. Thyme, a popular pizza spice, eliminates phlegm.[122] Garlic syrup is good for asthma attacks and garlic itself has been shown to lower blood pressure through actions of one of its components , methyl allyl trisulfide which dilates blood vessel walls.[123] The list of other herbs, that are usually not used as foods, and their cures is endless. Mullein is a pain killer and can induce sleep and[124] bilberry is said to improve one's night vision in a single dose. [125] Plantain, a common weed outside most doorsteps, can perform miracles in its humble state. Edward E. Shook, a reputed Herbalist tells the following story, "A lady whose arm was previously amputated due to abscessing (from a bee sting) came to see me...outside my door there was some plantain growing. I picked some of the leaves and gave them to the woman telling her to wash and crush them, make a poultice and apply it to the part where she had been stung. The next day this lady returned to thank me...the hand was entirely well."[126]

Furthermore, herbs do not just heal, help the body, and soothe, they can actually help to cure. Bernard Jensen reminds us in his book The Chemistry of Man that "we must realize that when we apply the mental, physical, mechanical and chemical therapies in the healing art, it will be to no avail if the nutritional foundation has not been properly laid." Herbs can be part of that foundation. Donald Lepore, ND, in his book The Ultimate Healing System, states that every vitamin, mineral and amino acid is available to one from an herbal source if we know where to look for it. [127] Honey, a common natural remedy, contains 35% protein and contains half of all the amino acids in a highly concentrated source as well as many essential nutrients.[128] Herbs nourish us while they heal us.

Natural therapies are the obvious complement to natural remedies. One reason the medical profession has such a low rate of accurate diagnosis of illness is because they are limited by their view of illness itself. The medical profession views illness as a problem that must be given a name so that then the name can be given a drug to make it go away. Natural therapists, on the other hand, see illness as a sign that the body is under stress and they look to the whole person for and answer to the "problem". They will evaluate the person's symptoms from their diet to their actual complaints and then recommend for them lifestyle changes as well as complementary herbs or homeopathic remedies to help their body recover more quickly. In the first case doctors are assuming they know more than our bodies and are giving our illness a name and then prescribing for that named illness. Natural therapists, on the other hand realize that, "It is more important what kind of person has the illness than what kind of illness the person has".[129] so rather than prescribing for a specific illness, they monitor the individual, giving them herbs to strengthen, nourish and help their body cure itself. With this method, knowing the name of the disease is not really important and in fact, irrelevant, as the body itself knows and when given the right herbs and nourishment can cure itself without us even having to know the name of the exact illness we had. In fact so many illnesses are so interrelated and similar, that it is becoming increasingly difficult to put a name on them anyway.

Natural therapies, besides looking at the whole person instead of just the charts and blood tests, also has many valuable tools for diagnosis that the medical profession do not use. Iridology, for example, has many advantages *over* any other form of diagnosis. The iridologist can determine inherent structure and working capacity of and organ, can detect environmental strain, can determine the nerve force, the responsive healing power of the tissue. Iridologists can see the condition of the colon in great detail, can spot potential tumors or problems in organs and can do all this and more simply by looking into the iris of the eye.

Most natural therapies also work *with* the individual's body rather than against their bodies. Massage, Reiki, Therapeutic Touch, Reflexology, Acupressure, Acupuncture and others focus their healing on giving positive energy to the body and stimulating the body's own healing points and capacity. Surgery, radiation and chemotherapy, on the other hand, although considered standard procedures for modern day cancer treatment - do nothing to restore the body's own protective organs and functions.[130]

The Eleventh Building Block of Health: Develop Self Awareness

- David Frohm, quoted in the book, <u>A Cancer Battle Plan,</u> written by his wife, Anne Frohm, describes this relationship beautifully when he tells her, *"Your body is like a garden God has given you to take care of...Now it is full of weeds (Her Cancer). Your job, until he reclaims the garden, is to do your best at getting rid of the weeds and growing the good stuff. Failure is not found in giving the garden back (dying), but in doing less than your best with it while it is yours."*[131]
- *"Eat and drink but waste not by excess for God loves not the prodigals"* (7:31 Koran)

The eleventh principal of health is to develop self-awareness. Wine is so forbidden in the Islam that the prophet said "Whosoever uses wine to treat his illness may God not give him recovery" (Hadith of the Prophet Muhammad) In the Koran chapter five, verse three, it says, Forbidden to you (for *food*) are: dead meat, blood, the flesh of swine, and that on which hath been invoked the name of other than Allah; that which hath been killed by strangling, or by a violent blow, or by a headlong fall, or by being gored to death; that which hath been (partly) eaten by a wild animal; unless ye are able to slaughter it (in due form); that which is sacrificed on stone (altars); (forbidden) also is the division (of meat) by raffling with arrows: that is

33

impiety... But if any is forced by hunger, with no inclination to transgression, Allah is indeed Oft-forgiving, Most Merciful." However, in Christianity this is not the same rule. In Mark chapter seven, verse nineteen it says, "since it enters, not his heart but his stomach, and so passes on?" (Thus he declared all foods clean.) "In Judaism there are strict laws of which foods are allowable and not allowable. In the Old Testament it says (Leviticus 11:47) to make a distinction between the unclean and the clean and between the living creature that may be eaten and the living creature that may not be eaten. These foods are called Kosher Foods. It is important to be aware of the guidelines God has laid out for you as well as to be aware of the other ways you are unique and differ from others. Our constitution, climates and available food sources are as varied as our beliefs. We cannot say that an Eskimo in Alaska should eat the same as a Japanese in Tokyo. We cannot say that there is just *one* right way of eating for everyone.

The Twelfth Building Block of Health: Knowledge

Wisdom of the Scriptures & Examples in Scriptures of the Virtues of Knowledge:
- *"Fast the month of Ramadan so that to heal your bodies from disease"* (Hadith)
- *"I will fetch my knowledge from afar, and ascribe righteousness to my Maker".* (Job 36:3: Bible)
- *"Teach me good judgment and knowledge, for I believe in thy commandments".* (Psalms 116:36: Bible)
- *"Oh my Lord, advance me in knowledge"* (20:114: Koran)
- *"For every Malady Allah created he also created its cure. Who acquires such knowledge shall benefit from it and one who ignores it will forgo such benefit."* (Sahih Bukhari: Muslim)

The twelfth principal of health and the "glue" that holds it all together is knowledge. Knowledge is our only armor in the battle of the advertisers. We are surrounded by companies telling us that their products are "nutritious" or "wholesome". We are bombarded with ads telling us the miracle of pharmaceuticals and we are buried in "information" the newspapers carry about the dangers of herbs or the quackery of homeopathy. Today even the natural health industry is flooded with companies selling substandard herbs which sometimes do not contain the correct forms of the herbs they claim to be selling, while other companies work hard to sell us their "super juice pills" or "super green drinks". Everyone is so convincing, and there are not any exact laws defining the words wholesome, natural and herbal, so the only way we can protect ourselves is to gain knowledge of how our bodies work and how they heal.

Not so long ago our scientists believed water to be an element and oxygen the cause of acidity, that Columbus discovered America[132], and the atom was the ultimate particle and the fly produced diseases. Recently eggs were thought to be bad for you, aspartame was popular, and high-protein diets were the rage for their rapid weight loss results. Of course all of these things have since gone out of style and been disproved. However, we are in the midst of more propaganda today. Vaccines, vitamins, milk chugs, and low fat foods are just a few of the fads that will soon pass (we hope!).The evidence against vaccines is overwhelming and it is only a matter of time before public protest will put a stop to them. In 1979, by a record count of inhabitants of the Philippines, out of 107,981 persons vaccinated, 59,000 died after vaccination.[133] The list of deaths, illnesses and other complications created by vaccines fills a number of books that are available on the market today and a growing number of parents are deciding not to vaccinate their children. One theory I have about vaccines is that they do not prevent illnesses, but simply suppress them so that instead of getting measles or mumps or chicken pox as a child we get asthma, cancer, AIDS and lupus (among others) as adults.

Vitamins are another fad that is slowly waning. People are beginning to realize that we have never and still are not aware of all the minerals and vitamins that exist. We are also realizing how complex the interrelationship between these vitamins and minerals is and the more we know the more difficult it becomes to properly combine vitamins. Only twenty years ago multi- vitamins made out of synthetic chemicals and containing standard doses of various vitamins were popular. Today, we are realizing that the organic human body cannot benefit from non-organic vitamins. We are also realizing that vitamins and minerals work together like a symphony in the body and that to take away and add one here and there without regard to the entire symphony would ruin the piece. We try to improve our orchestra by adding five violins only to find that they drown out the violas and may eliminate the flutes altogether. So we then add more flutes and violas only to have them drown out the violins and soon become bankrupt trying to repair the orchestra. Consumers are realizing that even natural vitamins are not a long-term solution (although short term therapeutic use has been proven effective in cases such as using vitamin C to combat colds and flus and speed healing or using vitamin B in times of stress), and that for long-term supplementation they either need to rely on their own good healthy eating habits or super foods and supplements made from them such as KyoGreen (BarleyGreen), FruitPlus Caps, and others.

In the past three years the "low fat" diet has been slowly losing ground as well. It has now been proven through the highly popularized Zone Diet that it is the carbohydrates that are our biggest villain in the weight loss game and that fat, in moderation is not only fine, but needed by the body as an efficient source of energy that carries the fat-soluble vitamins to the cells.[134]

Consumers need to gain knowledge about many things to protect themselves against today's and tomorrow's propaganda. They need to gain knowledge about herbs and natural therapies and especially about nutrition. Only seven out of sixty medical schools in the nation offer nutrition courses for their medical students so we can't rely on our doctors to help us eat right.[135] We need to know that white sugar leeches calcium from the body and causes a B-vitamin deficiency.[136] We need to know that yellow vegetables are laxatives, green vegetables are blood builders and red vegetable are arterial stimulants. We should know that drinking coffee an hour before a meal cuts iron absorption by 22%.[137] Perspiration can cause a loss of three times more potassium than sodium and cause a person to become allergic to everything. We should be aware that the blood is only as clean as the bowel and that the RDAs in general were charts created to keep the average young male away from nutrient related illnesses such as scurvy.[138]

We also need to educate ourselves about herbs. We read the labels and books and think we know everything but herbal secret are complex and only a professional would know the subtleties of the art and draw the line between safe herbs and unsafe self-prescribing. For instance, unripe capsules of the poppy contain many poisonous ions, while the seed of the same plant, when ripe contains a nutrient oil, but no poison.[139] If you combine herbs and foods such as iron and tannic acid this could result in death. Aloe, in large doses are poisonous, providing irritation of the intestinal wall, pain, vomiting, purging, cold sweats. prostration, convulsions and collapse.[140] Parsley can dry up mother's milk and senna tea should be drunk cold to prevent gripping.[141] These are just a few examples of herbal wisdom that are usually known only by experienced herbalist, the most important knowledge we need to gain is that disease is an elimination activity of the body.[142]

We are constantly fighting our bodies when we are ill and even when we are not ill. We need to learn to work with our bodies to produce health. In fact, all things that we try to squelch with over-the-counter medications actually have reasons. Pain is a warning that something is wrong. Fever inactivates many viruses and is our strongest weapon against bacteria, Mucus is produces in the respiratory tract to surround and carry off irritating material.[143] We need to work *with* our bodies and not against them to remain healthy and cure ourselves. We need to strengthen our relationship with God and ourselves, we need to eat whole raw and real foods, we need to be aware of how foods should be prepared, we need to drink pure water and breathe fresh air, we need to exercise and keep good hygiene and we need to turn to natural remedies and natural therapies. All diseases *are* curable, just not every patient[144] and instead of following the latest health fads, ads and media hype, we should remember what Marcel Proust said, "The real voyage of discovery consists not of seeking new lands but in seeing with new eyes."

Footnotes:
1 Cheraskin, E., MD, DMD, Ringsdorf, W.M. Jr., DMD, and Clark, J.W., DDS, Diet and Disease. Keats Publishing, 1968. Page 48.
2 Jensen, Bernard, Ph.D.., The Chemistry of Man. Bernard Jensen, 1983. Page 477.
3 Jensen, Bernard, Ph.D.., The Chemistry of Man. Bernard Jensen, 1983.
4 Krohn, Jacqueline, MD, The Whole Way to Allergy Relief and Prevention. Hartley and Marks, 1991. Page 8.
5 Corp of the President of The Church of Jesus Christ of Latter-day Saints Book of Mormon© 1981 Page 194.
6 http://www.azamra.org/heal/hezekiah.html link
7 Jensen, Bernard, DC, Ph.D.., The Science and Practice of Iridology Volume I. Bernard Jensen International, 1995. Page 187.
8 Morter, Dr. Ted M. Jr., MA, Your Health...Your Choice. Lifetime Books Inc., 1995. Page 29.
9 Oyle, Dr. Irving, The Healing Mind. NA. Page 9.

10 Hoffer, Abram, MD, Ph.D.., and Walker, Morton, DPM, Putting it all Together: The New Orthomolecular Nutrition. Keats Publishing, 1978. Page 49.

11 Hoffer, Abram, MD, Ph.D.., and Walker, Morton, DPM, Putting it all Together: The New Orthomolecular Nutrition. Keats Publishing, 1978. Page 32.

12 Jensen, Bernard, Ph.D.., The Chemistry of Man. Bernard Jensen, 1983. Page 474.

13 Jensen, Bernard, Ph.D.., The Chemistry of Man. Bernard Jensen, 1983. Page 276.

14 Jensen, Bernard, Ph.D.., The Chemistry of Man. Bernard Jensen, 1983. Page 191.

15 Lepore, Donald, ND, The Ultimate Healing System. Lepore, 1985. Page 294.

16 Frahm, Anne E. and David J., A Cancer Battle Plan. Tarcher & Putnam Press, 1992. Page 113.

17 Jensen, Bernard, DC, Ph.D.., The Science and Practice of Iridology Volume I. Bernard Jensen International, 1995. Page 151.

18 Jensen, Bernard, Ph.D.., The Chemistry of Man. Bernard Jensen, 1983. Page 32.

19 Jensen, Bernard, Ph.D.., The Chemistry of Man. Bernard Jensen, 1983. Page 150.

20 Jensen, Bernard, Ph.D.., The Chemistry of Man. Bernard Jensen, 1983. Page 70.

21 Jensen, Bernard, Ph.D.., The Chemistry of Man. Bernard Jensen, 1983. Page 23.

22 Oyle, Dr. Irving, The Healing Mind. NA. Page 48.

23 Oyle, Dr. Irving, The Healing Mind. NA. Pages 1,2 &8.

24 Corp of the President of The Church of Jesus Christ of Latter-day Saints Doctrine & Covenants© 1981

25 Hoffer, Abram, MD, Ph.D.., and Walker, Morton, DPM, Putting it all Together: The New Orthomolecular Nutrition. Keats Publishing, 1978. Page 18.

26 Hoffer, Abram, MD, Ph.D.., and Walker, Morton, DPM, Putting it all Together: The New Orthomolecular Nutrition. Keats Publishing, 1978. Page 5.

27 Jensen, Bernard, Ph.D.., The Chemistry of Man. Bernard Jensen, 1983. Page 381.

28 Jensen, Bernard, Ph.D.., The Chemistry of Man. Bernard Jensen, 1983. Page 235.

29 Cheraskin, E., MD, DMD, Ringsdorf, W.M. Jr., DMD, and Clark, J.W., DDS, Diet and Disease. Keats Publishing, 1968. Page 18.

30 Morter, Dr. Ted M. Jr., MA, Your Health...Your Choice. Lifetime Books Inc., 1995. Page 142.

31 Hoffer, Abram, MD, Ph.D.., and Walker, Morton, DPM, Putting it all Together: The New Orthomolecular Nutrition. Keats Publishing, 1978. Page 84.

32 Morter, Dr. Ted M. Jr., MA, Your Health...Your Choice. Lifetime Books Inc., 1995. Page 217.

33 Jensen, Bernard, DC, Ph.D.., The Science and Practice of Iridology Volume I. Bernard Jensen International, 1995. Page 103.

34 Jensen, Bernard, Ph.D.., The Chemistry of Man. Bernard Jensen, 1983. Page 50.

35 Morter, Dr. Ted M. Jr., MA, Your Health...Your Choice. Lifetime Books Inc., 1995. Page 58.

36 Note that Old Testament quotes apply to Jewish and Christian faith.

37 Frahm, Anne E. and David J., A Cancer Battle Plan. Tarcher & Putnam Press, 1992. Page 82.

38 Krohn, Jacqueline, MD, The Whole Way to Allergy Relief and Prevention. Hartley and Marks, 1991. Page 62.

39 Morter, Dr. Ted M. Jr., MA, Your Health...Your Choice. Lifetime Books Inc., 1995. Page 74.

40 Jensen, Bernard, DC, Ph.D.., The Science and Practice of Iridology Volume I. Bernard Jensen International, 1995. Page 168.

41 Krohn, Jacqueline, MD, The Whole Way to Allergy Relief and Prevention. Hartley and Marks, 1991. Page 107.

42 Jensen, Bernard, DC, Ph.D.., The Science and Practice of Iridology Volume I. Bernard Jensen International, 1995.

43 Morter, Dr. Ted M. Jr., MA, Your Health...Your Choice. Lifetime Books Inc., 1995. Page 211.

44 Krohn, Jacqueline, MD, The Whole Way to Allergy Relief and Prevention. Hartley and Marks, 1991. Page 7.

45 Morter, Dr. Ted M. Jr., MA, Your Health...Your Choice. Lifetime Books Inc., 1995. Page 181.

46 Jensen, Bernard, Ph.D.., The Chemistry of Man. Bernard Jensen, 1983. Page 9.

47 Hoffer, Abram, MD, Ph.D.., and Walker, Morton, DPM, Putting it all Together: The New Orthomolecular Nutrition. Keats Publishing, 1978. Page 18.

48 Romano, Rita, Dining in the Raw. Kensington Books, 1992. Page 15.

49 Romano, Rita, Dining in the Raw. Kensington Books, 1992. Page 15.

50 48 Hours Special Report 7/14/99

51 Morter, Dr. Ted M. Jr., MA, Your Health...Your Choice. Lifetime Books Inc., 1995. Page 37.

52 Balch, James F., MD and Phyllis A., CNC, Prescription for Nutritional Healing Second Edition. Avery Press, 1997. Page 47.

53 Jensen, Bernard, Ph.D.., The Chemistry of Man. Bernard Jensen, 1983. Page 178.

54 Morter, Dr. Ted M. Jr., MA, Your Health...Your Choice. Lifetime Books Inc., 1995. Page 166.

55 Hoffer, Abram, MD, Ph.D.., and Walker, Morton, DPM, Putting it all Together: The New Orthomolecular Nutrition. Keats Publishing, 1978. Page 9.

56 Tierra, Michael, CA, ND. Planetary Herbology. Lotus Press, 1988. Page 80.

57 Tierra, Michael, CA, ND. Planetary Herbology. Lotus Press, 1988. Page 77.

58 Tierra, Michael, CA, ND. Planetary Herbology. Lotus Press, 1988. Page 74.

59 Jensen, Bernard, Ph.D.., The Chemistry of Man. Bernard Jensen, 1983.

60 Jensen, Bernard, Ph.D.., The Chemistry of Man. Bernard Jensen, 1983. Page 40.

61 Jensen, Bernard, Ph.D.., The Chemistry of Man. Bernard Jensen, 1983. Page 384.

62 Morter, Dr. Ted M. Jr., MA, Your Health...Your Choice. Lifetime Books Inc., 1995. Page 207.

63 Jensen, Bernard, Ph.D.., The Chemistry of Man. Bernard Jensen, 1983. Page 17.

64 Morter, Dr. Ted M. Jr., MA, Your Health...Your Choice. Lifetime Books Inc., 1995. Page 119.

65 Jensen, Bernard, Ph.D.., The Chemistry of Man. Bernard Jensen, 1983. Page 34.

66 Jensen, Bernard, Ph.D.., The Chemistry of Man. Bernard Jensen, 1983. Page 197.

67 Lepore, Donald, ND, The Ultimate Healing System. Lepore, 1985. Page 10.

68 Jensen, Bernard, DC, Ph.D.., The Science and Practice of Iridology Volume I. Bernard Jensen International, 1995. Page 336.

69 Jensen, Bernard, Ph.D.., The Chemistry of Man. Bernard Jensen, 1983. Page 40.

70 Frahm, Anne E. and David J., A Cancer Battle Plan. Tarcher & Putnam Press, 1992. Page 79.

71 Morter, Dr. Ted M. Jr., MA, Your Health…Your Choice. Lifetime Books Inc., 1995. Page 225.

72 Morter, Dr. Ted M. Jr., MA, Your Health…Your Choice. Lifetime Books Inc., 1995. Page 225.

73 Morter, Dr. Ted M. Jr., MA, Your Health…Your Choice. Lifetime Books Inc., 1995. Page 221.

74 Hoffer, Abram, MD, Ph.D.., and Walker, Morton, DPM, Putting it all Together: The New Orthomolecular Nutrition. Keats Publishing, 1978. Page 89.

75 Morter, Dr. Ted M. Jr., MA, Your Health…Your Choice. Lifetime Books Inc., 1995. Page 27.

76 Morter, Dr. Ted M. Jr., MA, Your Health…Your Choice. Lifetime Books Inc., 1995. Page 119.

77 Morter, Dr. Ted M. Jr., MA, Your Health…Your Choice. Lifetime Books Inc., 1995. Page 119.

78 Morter, Dr. Ted M. Jr., MA, Your Health…Your Choice. Lifetime Books Inc., 1995. Page 83.

79 Balch, James F., MD and Phyllis A., CNC, Prescription for Nutritional Healing Second Edition.

80 Note that in all passages the reference is to "walk with God" and not "sit with God."

81 Akili, Imam Muhammad, Medicine of the Prophet, Pearl Publishing House 1994. Page 191.

82 Jensen, Bernard, DC, Ph.D.., The Science and Practice of Iridology Volume I. Bernard Jensen International, 1995. Page 84.

83 Krohn, Jacqueline, MD, The Whole Way to Allergy Relief and Prevention. Hartley and Marks, 1991.

84 Jensen, Bernard, DC, Ph.D.., The Science and Practice of Iridology Volume I. Bernard Jensen International, 1995. Page 171.

85 Krohn, Jacqueline, MD, The Whole Way to Allergy Relief and Prevention. Hartley and Marks, 1991.

Page 263.

86 Morter, Dr. Ted M. Jr., MA, Your Health...Your Choice. Lifetime Books Inc., 1995. Page 235.

87 Morter, Dr. Ted M. Jr., MA, Your Health...Your Choice. Lifetime Books Inc., 1995. Page 63.

88 Frahm, Anne E. and David J., A Cancer Battle Plan. Tarcher & Putnam Press, 1992. Page 85.

89 Take note in the following passages that purity is associated with water in general and that the word breathe is used synonymously with the word life.

90 Balch, James F., MD and Phyllis A., CNC, Prescription for Nutritional Healing Second Edition. Avery Press, 1997. Pages 3 & 30.

91 Shook, Edward E., ND, DC, Advance Treatise in Herbology. Wendell Whitman Company. Page 318.

92 Balch, James F., MD and Phyllis A., CNC, Prescription for Nutritional Healing Second Edition. Avery Press, 1997. Page 30.

93 Jensen, Bernard, Ph.D.., The Chemistry of Man. Bernard Jensen, 1983. Page 70.

94 Lepore, Donald, ND, The Ultimate Healing System. Lepore, 1985. Page 57.

95 Balch, James F., MD and Phyllis A., CNC, Prescription for Nutritional Healing Second Edition. Avery Press, 1997. Page 32.

96 Jensen, Bernard, Ph.D.., The Chemistry of Man. Bernard Jensen, 1983. Page 165.

97 Lepore, Donald, ND, The Ultimate Healing System. Lepore, 1985. Page 340.

98 Jensen, Bernard, Ph.D.., The Chemistry of Man. Bernard Jensen, 1983. Page 258.

99 Jensen, Bernard, Ph.D.., The Chemistry of Man. Bernard Jensen, 1983. Page 10.

100 Krohn, Jacqueline, MD, The Whole Way to Allergy Relief and Prevention. Hartley and Marks, 1991.

101 Shook, Edward E., ND, DC, Advance Treatise in Herbology. Wendell Whitman Company. Page 42.

102 Jensen, Bernard, Ph.D.., The Chemistry of Man. Bernard Jensen, 1983. Page 364.

103 Shook, Edward E., ND, DC, Advance Treatise in Herbology. Wendell Whitman Company. Page 102.

104 Schumacher, Teresa, Cleansing the Body and the Colon for a Happier and Healthier You. 1997.

105 Shook, Edward E., ND, DC, Advance Treatise in Herbology. Wendell Whitman Company. Page 31.

106 Kristie Burns

107 Shook, Edward E., ND, DC, Advance Treatise in Herbology. Wendell Whitman Company. Page 21.

108 Lepore, Donald, ND, The Ultimate Healing System. Lepore, 1985. Page 78.

109 Panos, Maesimund B., MD, and Heimlich, Jane, Homeopathic Medicine at Home. Tarcher & Putnam, 1980. Page 132.

110 Lepore, Donald, ND, The Ultimate Healing System. Lepore, 1985. Page 130.

111 Shook, Edward E., ND, DC, Advance Treatise in Herbology. Wendell Whitman Company. Page 81.

112 Jensen, Bernard, DC, Ph.D.., The Science and Practice of Iridology Volume I. Bernard Jensen International, 1995/ Page 13.

113 Graedon, Teresa and Joe, Deadly Drug Interactions: The People's Pharmacy Guide. St. Martin's Press 1997.

114 Oyle, Dr. Irving, The Healing Mind. NA. Page 11.

115 Oyle, Dr. Irving, The Healing Mind. NA. Page 10.

116 Oyle, Dr. Irving, The Healing Mind. NA. Page 11.

117 Jensen, Bernard, DC, Ph.D.., The Science and Practice of Iridology Volume I. Bernard Jensen International, 1995. Page 23.

118 Jensen, Bernard, DC, Ph.D.., The Science and Practice of Iridology Volume I. Bernard Jensen International, 1995. Page 23.

119 Shook, Edward E., ND, DC, Advance Treatise in Herbology. Wendell Whitman Company. Page 182.

120 Balch, James F., MD and Phyllis A., CNC, Prescription for Nutritional Healing Second Edition. Avery Press, 1997. Page 62-3.

121 Pederson, Mark, Nutritional Herbology. Wendell Whitman Company, 1987. Page 129.

122 Buchman, Dian Dincin, Herbal Medicine. Wings Books, 1996.

123 Balch, James F., MD and Phyllis A., CNC, Prescription for Nutritional Healing Second Edition. Avery Press, 1997. Page 54.

124 Lepore, Donald, ND, The Ultimate Healing System. Lepore, 1985. Page 186.

125 Pederson, Mark, Nutritional Herbology. Wendell Whitman Company, 1987. Page 46.

126 Shook, Edward E., ND, DC, Advance Treatise in Herbology. Wendell Whitman Company. Page 40.

127 Lepore, Donald, ND, The Ultimate Healing System. Lepore, 1985. Page 135.

128 Balch, James F., MD and Phyllis A., CNC, Prescription for Nutritional Healing Second Edition. Avery Press, 1997. Page 55.

129 Jensen, Bernard, Ph.D.., The Chemistry of Man. Bernard Jensen, 1983. Page 28.

130 Frahm, Anne E. and David J., A Cancer Battle Plan. Tarcher & Putnam Press, 1992. Page 40.

131 Frahm, Anne E. and David J., A Cancer Battle Plan. Tarcher & Putnam Press, 1992. Page 112.

132 Petit, Charles W., Rediscovering America. US News & World Report, October 12, 1998.

133 Jensen, Bernard, DC, Ph.D.., The Science and Practice of Iridology Volume I. Bernard Jensen International, 1995. Page 117.

134 Jensen, Bernard, Ph.D.., The Chemistry of Man. Bernard Jensen, 1983. Page 29.

135 Jensen, Bernard, Ph.D.., The Chemistry of Man. Bernard Jensen, 1983. Page 371.

136 Jensen, Bernard, Ph.D.., The Chemistry of Man. Bernard Jensen, 1983. Page 30.

137 Jensen, Bernard, Ph.D.., The Chemistry of Man. Bernard Jensen, 1983. Page 95.

138 Hoffer, Abram, MD, Ph.D.., and Walker, Morton, DPM, Putting it all Together: The New Orthomolecular Nutrition. Keats Publishing, 1978. Page 10.

139 Shook, Edward E., ND, DC, Advance Treatise in Herbology. Wendell Whitman Company. Page 137.

140 Shook, Edward E., ND, DC, Advance Treatise in Herbology. Wendell Whitman Company. Page 219.

141 Lepore, Donald, ND, The Ultimate Healing System. Lepore, 1985. Page 199.

142 Jensen, Bernard, DC, Ph.D.., The Science and Practice of Iridology Volume I. Bernard Jensen International, 1995. Page 35.

143 Panos, Maesimund B., MD, and Heimlich, Jane, Homeopathic Medicine at Home. Tarcher & Putnam, 1980. Page 14.

144 Jensen, Bernard, DC, Ph.D.., The Science and Practice of Iridology Volume I. Bernard Jensen International, 1995. Page 43.

Assignment for Section One

Imagine you were going to change this article to talk about the "13" principles of health instead of 12. What would you add to this list and why? Your "addition" to this article should be at least 3 paragraphs long and should include references (either books, magazines or online sources).

~Section Two: Modern Nutritional Dangers~

I have always maintained that it did not make sense for something created by nature to be unhealthy. This is what all religions, spiritual medicine and logic teach. Eggs were a natural food in the most pure unaltered sense of the definition. As long as they were eaten in moderation (spiritual guides from all religions recommend moderation) and they were natural (another spiritual constant in all religions) that they were good. That was in 1986. Now, starting in 1998, studies started being published that show that not only are eggs good for you that they are necessary for the brain development of children and not only that – that the white part of the egg contains a substance that cancels out the harmful cholesterol in the yellow part of the egg. Others can wait for the studies to come out on the following items. For me, I rely on the more timeless wisdom of moderation and nature. In this chapter I have covered alcohol, alkaline imbalance, aluminum, aspartame & MSG, bread & carbohydrate addiction, chlorine & fluoride, coffee, dietary supplements and vitamins, colloidal silver, cow's milk, soda pop, sodium laurel sulfate & other chemicals, tobacco, and excess bread.

Alcohol
As far as the body is concerned, alcohol is a poison. Some of the effects of alcohol are damage to the brain, liver, pancreas, duodenum and central nervous system. It causes metabolic damage to every cell in the body. The only studies done on healthful uses of alcohol involve a highly publicized study on red wine consumption in France which showed lower cholesterol levels and healthy in people drinking red wine daily. This may be true for those people who drank red wine daily and also ate a whole foods diet (as most of the people in the study did). However, how many people who drink only red wine, drink only 1-2 glasses with a meal and also eat a whole foods diet devoid of packaged and sugared foods? At the same time scientists have isolated the factor in red wine, which makes it healthy. It is grape seed. This herb is readily available in the herbal extract from any store and much safer than wine. Recent studies have even shown that cocoa has more antioxidants than wine!

Alcohol causes metabolic damage to every cell in the body in a slow insidious way so that it may take years for one to actually notice the damage. The liver, which is the ONLY organ which processes the alcohol, can actually be up to 3/4 damaged before it shuts down. That is why liver disease is so hard to detect early.

When alcohol is broken down in the liver it inhibits the liver's production of digestive enzymes and impairs the body's ability to absorb fats, proteins and the fat soluble vitamins (A, D, E, and K) as well as the B-complex vitamins. Because of the work the liver must do to process the alcohol, toxic amounts of fat get stuck in the liver. And while the liver can usually regenerate itself (up to 25% can be removed and it will grow back within three months), alcohol actually destroys this ability to some extent and some liver damage caused by alcohol can never be reversed.

Another common effect of alcohol on the body of the regular consumer is that of damage to the PERIPHERAL nervous system. This means the feet and hands. One may experience shaking or loss of sensation in either. The pancreas also becomes inflamed and this can lead to diabetes. Men who drink alcohol experience a great decrease in their production of testosterone, a male hormone which is basically responsible for making them: "male". Alcohol is also one of the most common causes of reduced sexual performance, impotence and infertility.

People consuming large amounts of alcohol may also eventually become deficient in zinc which can cause one to lose their sense of taste or smell and thus some of their enjoyment of food. This also impairs their ability to heal wounds so alcoholics who get injured or have surgical scars may never heal properly.

Combining alcohol with over the counter drugs like Panadol, Tylenol and others has often proved deadly to some people. If you are allergic to suphites (sulpha drugs, sulphites, etc.) then alcohol is even more deadly for you as it is manufactured with sulphites. Children of people who are addicted to alcohol often find themselves addicts of substances as well. They may become addicted to food (obesity), to smoking (cigarettes) or even video games or sugar.

Symptoms directly related to a drinking problem would be: dizziness, delayed reflexes, slowed mental function, memory loss, poor judgment, emotional outbursts, aggressive behavior, lack of coordination, shaking of the hands, nervous system disorders and anxiety. Symptoms of withdrawal (when trying to quit) are: craving, nausea, vomiting, gastrointestinal upset, abdominal cramps, anorexia, fatigue, headache, anxiety, irritability, chills, depression, insomnia, tremors, weakness and hallucinations.

Alkaline Imbalance

One of the strongest basis of natural healing WORLDWIDE (think Thai Medicine, Chinese Medicine, Ayurveda, Islamic Medicine, etc.) is balance. This balance is seen in the body by Avicenna as a balance of the four humors. In modern medicine this balance is measured with blood tests that should read a certain number to qualify as "balanced". Don't disregard a method of diagnosis just because it is not inside the traditional realm of your chosen healing system. There are many ways to see imbalance in the body. And as long as you know what to do to correct these imbalances you can view the body in that way. Keep in mind that HOW you evaluate a client will have a lot to do with how you help them and educate them. For example, a doctor may evaluate a patient's cholesterol levels with machines and get numbers as a result. The outcome of a cure must then follow the same rules. The doctor must then prescribe a medicine based on numbers and calculations specific to that number of imbalance in the system.

In the case of natural healing, when you evaluate a client by humeral imbalance you must then do something to balance those humors. For example if they have a runny nose you may view them as having excess phlegmatic humor and you would help them find an herb or natural method to expel excess phlegm from the body. In the same way you can use other methods to help people learn more about their bodies.

One useful marker for "general imbalance" in the body is the alkaline-acid level in the body. This is not as specific as detecting humeral imbalance but it can be a useful preparation for deeper healing and I find it a useful tool to clean out the body and prepare someone for deeper evaluation. It is like trying to clean a room. If everything is in a pile it may look impossible but if you can sort everything into boxes first and throw out some of the surface garbage it may be easier to see under the surface and get the job done more efficiently. This is what balancing the alkaline and acid levels in the body means to me.

Detecting the imbalance can be done with Ph papers or chemical tests or even urinalysis. There are some who say that the darker the color of the urine, the more acidic it is. Clearer urine indicates a more balanced system. I also look at a person's irises. If the iris is clear and not cloudy then the person is balanced. Over-acidity shows up in the iris as a "white tinge" to the spokes of the iris. Everything looks like it is whitish in color. This is an indication of an over acidic body.

Over acidity, which can become a dangerous condition that weakens all body systems, is very common today. It gives rise to an internal environment conducive to disease, as opposed to a pH- balanced environment which allows normal body function necessary for the body to resist disease. A healthy body maintains adequate alkaline reserves to meet emergency demands. When access acids must be neutralized our alkaline reserves are depleted leaving the body in a weakened condition. The concept of acid alkaline imbalance as the cause of disease is not new. In 1933 a New York doctor named William Howard Hay published a ground-breaking book, *A New Health Era* in which he maintains that all disease is caused by **autotoxication** (or "self-poisoning") due to acid accumulation in the body.

Aluminum

The subject of aluminum toxicity has caused controversy for at least twenty years and has been known to be toxic for over a hundred years (depending on amounts.) It is found in our food supply, in the air and soil, and is bound to bauxite in nature. Only in the last thirty years or so have we been exposed to it in such quantities because of processed food, metal tins, water supply and hygiene products.

You'll be surprised to learn some of the offending substances where we find fairly large quantities of added aluminum. Sliced cheese singles, many other dairy products as an emulsifier, infant formula, cake mixes, baking powder, self-rising flour, commercial dough, non-dairy creamer, pickles, dandruff shampoo (Selsun Blue,) and, of course, anti-perspirants and antacids.

In nonfood items, it's in every can of pop and beer, most cookware, most major city water supplies used to settle out solids, and is in the from pollution. Some countries have very high levels because of spent mines. Recently, an old mineshaft in West Virginia broke open and water, sludge and tailings roared down the mountainside, fouling the area with one of the worst environmental disasters in a long time. It gets into the groundwater system through agriculture from soil erosion and poor current mining practices.

Aspartame & MSG

Aspartame and other man-made sweeteners are unnecessary and dangerous for the body. The guideline for this knowledge, is of course, that they are not natural at all. Even sweeteners extracted from plants are not natural because they have been extracted from the plant in an unnatural way and are separated from the minerals and vitamins that help one digest the complete food. There are even plants, such as stevia, which are found in nature and provide perfect substitutes for sugar. And pure dried cane juice has only a percentage of the problems that white sugar does so even switching to pure dried cane would be a dietary improvement. There is no reason to resort to unnatural chemicals when nature has provided us already with solutions.

Aspartame is the technical name for the brand names, NutraSweet, Equal, Spoonful, and Equal- Measure. Aspartame was discovered by accident in 1965, when James Schlatter, a chemist of G.D. Searle Company was testing an anti-ulcer drug. Aspartame was approved for dry goods in 1981 and for carbonated beverages in 1983. It was originally approved for dry goods on July 26, 1974, but objections filed by neuroscience researcher Dr John W. Olney and Consumer attorney James Turner in August 1974 as well as investigations of G.D. Searle's research practices caused the US Food and Drug Administration (FDA) to put approval of aspartame on hold (December 5, 1974). In 1985, Monsanto purchased G.D. Searle and made Searle Pharmaceuticals and The NutraSweet Company separate subsidiaries.

Aspartame accounts for over 75 percent of the adverse reactions to food additives reported to the US Food and Drug Administration (FDA). Many of these reactions are very serious including seizures and death as recently disclosed in a February 1994 Department of Health and Human Services report.(1) A few of the 90 different documented symptoms listed in the report as being caused by aspartame include: Headaches/migraines, dizziness, seizures, nausea, numbness, muscle spasms, weight gain, rashes, depression, fatigue, irritability, tachycardia, insomnia, vision problems, hearing loss, heart palpitations, breathing difficulties, anxiety attacks, slurred speech, loss of taste, tinnitus, vertigo, memory loss, and joint pain.

According to researchers and physicians studying the adverse effects of aspartame, the following chronic illnesses can be triggered or worsened by ingesting of aspartame:(2) Brain tumors, multiple sclerosis, epilepsy, chronic fatigue syndrome, parkinson's disease, alzheimer's, mental retardation, lymphoma, birth defects, fibromyalgia, and diabetes. Aspartame is made up of three chemicals: Aspartic acid, phenylalanine, and methanol. The book, **Prescription for Nutritional Healing**, by James and Phyllis Balch, lists aspartame under the category of "chemical poison." As you shall see, that is exactly what it is. ASPARTIC ACID (40% OF ASPARTAME) Dr Russell L. Blaylock, a professor of Neurosurgery at the Medical University of Mississippi, recently published a book thoroughly detailing the damage that is caused by the ingestion of excessive aspartic acid from aspartame. Ninety nine percent of monosodium glutamate 9MSG) is glutamic acid. The damage it causes is also documented in Blaylock's book.] Blaylock makes use of almost 500 scientific references to show how excess free excitatory amino acids such as aspartic acid and glutamic acid in our food supply are causing serious chronic neurological disorders and a myriad of other acute symptoms.(3) Aspartate and glutamate (MSG) act as neurotransmitters in the brain by facilitating the transmission of information from neuron to neuron. Too much aspartate or glutamate in the brain kills certain neurons by allowing the influx of too much calcium into the cells. This influx triggers excessive amounts of free radicals which kill the cells. The neural cell damage that can be caused by excessive aspartate and glutamate is why they are referred to as "excitotoxins." be caused by excessive aspartate and glutamate is why they are referred to as "excitotoxins." They "excite" or stimulate the neural cells to death. Aspartic acid is an amino acid. Taken in its free form (unbound to proteins) it significantly raises the blood plasma level of aspartate and glutamate. The excess aspartate and glutamate in the blood plasma shortly after ingesting aspartame or products with free glutamic acid (glutamate precursor) leads to a high level of those neurotransmitters in certain areas of the brain.

The blood brain barrier (BBB) which normally protects the brain from excess glutamate and aspartate as well as toxins 1) is not fully developed during childhood, 2) does not fully protect all areas of the brain, 3) is damaged by numerous chronic and acute conditions, and 4) allows seepage of excess glutamate and aspartate into the brain even when intact. The excess glutamate and aspartate slowly begin to destroy neurons. The large majority (75%+) of neural cells in a particular area of the brain are killed before any clinical symptoms of a chronic illness are noticed. A few of the many chronic illnesses that have been shown to be contributed to by long-term exposure excitatory amino acid damage include: Multiple sclerosis (MS), ALS, memory loss, hormonal problems, hearing loss, epilepsy, Alzheimer's disease, Parkinson's disease, hypoglycemia, AIDS dementia, brain lessions, and neuroendocrine disorders.

Bread & Carbohydrate Addiction

Traditional nutritional healing all the way back to Hippocrates teaches that everything can be harmful in excess – even bread. It also emphasizes the balance of the humors through proper food combining. Thus, it should come as no surprise that over-consumption of bread and other carbohydrates can be harmful to the health. As many as seventy-five percent of those who are overweight, and many normal-weight individuals as well, are carbohydrate addicted. Though many people may suspect there is a physical imbalance that makes them crave carbohydrates and put weight on easily, the underlying cause of their cravings and weight struggles often goes undiagnosed and untreated.

Carbohydrate addiction is caused by an imbalance - an over release of the hormone, insulin, when carbohydrate-rich foods are eaten. Among its many jobs, insulin signals the body to take in food (it has been called the "hunger hormone") and, once the food is consumed, signals the body to store the food energy in the form of fat. Too much insulin results in too strong an impulse to eat, too often, and a body that too readily stores food in the form of fat.

The scientific term for this condition is *post-prandial reactive hyperinsulinemia* which means too much insulin is released after eating. Over time, people who are hyperinsulinemic become insulin resistant, that is, the cells in their muscles, nervous systems, and organs start to close down to the high levels of insulin in their blood. Insulin is no longer able to open the doors to these cells and allow food energy (blood sugar or glucose) to enter. At this point, one may experience symptoms of low-blood sugar levels (hypoglycemia) including irritability, shakiness, **tiredness**, intense cravings, confusion, and headaches. Since the blood sugar cannot easily enter the muscles, nervous system, or organs, much of the food energy gets channeled into the fat cells and weight gain comes easily. Over time, however, as high insulin levels continue, even the fat cells can shut down and the blood glucose gets trapped in the blood stream bringing on the condition known as adult-onset diabetes.

However, aside from carbohydrates in general, wheat also has its own problems in excess. And sometimes even in normal amounts. Following the guideline of Islamic medicine that one should eat food from what grows in their region, we can see why so many people today have allergies or trouble digesting wheat. For the wheat that is grown and distributed today on a wide scale is called 'Spring Wheat" it is only one variety of the possible 3000 that used to be known. There is now an effort to bring back some alternative wheat such as spelt and kamut and this is a good thing. But one wonders if we can ever undo the damage that was done by completely wiping out thousands of years of wheat diversity and replacing it with one or two varieties which we expect the entire earth to consume.

Additionally, the kind of wheat that is on the market today, when consumed in excess (more than one serving a day) can leach iron from the system. This is perhaps one reason so many "bread addicts" are tired all the time.

"Now we depart from health in just the proportion to which we have allowed our alkalies to be dissipated by introduction of acid-forming food in too great amount... It may seem strange to say that all disease is the same thing, no matter what its myriad modes of expression, but it is verily so." William Howard Hay, M.D.

More recently, in his remarkable book Alkalizer Diet (see recommended reading), Dr. Theodore A. Baroody says essentially the same thing: *The countless names of illnesses do not really matter. What does matter is that they all come from the same root cause...too much tissue acid waste in the body! Theodore A. Baroody, N.D., D.C., Ph.D.*

Chlorine & Fluoride

Chlorine and fluoride, of course, are not recommended for use for the same reasons that colloidal silver is not recommended. It is natural but it is toxic in even small amounts. Much water pollution today results from the run-off from fields, which have been sprayed with insecticides and chemical fertilizers. Fluoride and chlorine are two other predominate pollutants in today's water supply. Fluoride has been shown to have numerous serious effects on the human body, including being carcinogenic. At 15 ppm (parts per million), it will destroy cellular enzyme systems. Chlorine has been shown to cause cardiovascular disease. Some people feel that by using bottled water they are avoiding this problem. However, chlorine is in our bath water and swimming pools and one can absorb approximately 5 times as much chlorine through your skin in a 10-minute shower as you would by drinking 5 cups of tap water. Chlorine is a powerful free radical that can cause damage to all living tissue.

Coffee and Caffeine

Caffeine, sugar and nicotine all stimulate the adrenal glands and thus weaken them with persistent and chronic use. A cycle is then created. You weaken the adrenal glands with the consumption of caffeine (and sugar and nicotine make it even worse), then your body in turn CRAVES these things to give it a pick-me-up for the fatigue you have created. It is a vicious cycle.

Caffeine is a member of the methylxanthine chemicals and drugs and stimulates the central nervous system. Initially, caffeine may lower blood sugar but then it leads to increased hunger and cravings for sweets for after adrenal stimulation blood sugar rises again. Caffeine also increases respiratory rates so people who have breathing problems may be attracted to it for that reason despite the horrible side effects. It is also a mild laxative so you will find people who drink coffee have good elimination even if their digestive system is not really functioning well the coffee and caffeine will give an illusion of function by helping them keep up regular and perhaps even very frequent bowel movements (3-6 a day is not uncommon when a caffeine or coffee consumer has become overloaded with the product).

The acid in coffee eats away at the vili of the small intestine reducing the nutrient assimilation ability of the intestines. So whatever nutrients are left after the coffee depletes some are not assimilated well anyway. For this reason caffeine consumers are usually deficient in calcium as well as other minerals. Calcium is a mineral which supports bone integrity, healthy teeth and a calm nervous system. People who are lacking in calcium may show signs of anxiety, osteoporosis and/or tooth decay and shaking of the hands or twitching in the face. There are further problems for specific beverages. Tea contains tannic acid which is a diuretic for potassium which means it can leach potassium from the body thus weakening the heart and causing anxiety or heart disease. There are several basis for concern with coffee drinking in particular. The easily rancified oils used in processing and the irritating acids contained in the beans themselves offer hazards beyond the caffeine itself.

The amount of caffeine needed for stimulation INCREASES with regular use as is typical of all addictive drugs. We all know this if we have used coffee before and yet we deceive ourselves into thinking it "must be OK because the government has not outlawed it yet". In fact, many countries have outlawed coffee during different periods in their history...and come on now - how many of you using that excuse really have that much faith in the government's ability to protect you from harm anyway?

Another thought we console ourselves with is the thought that "practically everyone drinks coffee - right? And they're OK"....now think about that one again. Think of all the people you know who drink a lot of caffeine and then list the problems they have. You will find that this statement is not true although it is easy to say and think. Furthermore the same people who find this statement so easy to say are the same people who may also sit around criticizing humanity in general for not being good, wise or smart or efficient or honest enough. So...you have to choose - do you think everyone around you is just so perfectly smart that they know what is good for them and for you or do you stick with your original thoughts and suspicions that "humanity really does need some more education" :) ...?

Further bad news is that caffeine consumption creates a need in your body for manganese and copper, and yet it supplies neither of these minerals. The diuretic effects of caffeine also lead to a lot of urinary loss of nutrients. In the same way that increased use of "diet water pills" can hurt you, caffeine can do the same by causing your body to leach itself of minerals and nutrients it needs.

The good news is that caffeine addiction is one of the easier addictions to cure and can still be used in moderation after the "cure". The following side effects are caused by caffeine consumption that is higher than 1 cup a day (or two sodas or teas a day):
- Excess nervousness, irritability, insomnia, dizziness and fatigue
- Headaches
- Heartburn
- General anxiety and panic attacks
- Hyperactivity (and bed wetting in children)
- Increased stomach hydrochloric acid production
- Loss of minerals such as potassium, magnesium, zinc, and vitamins including B and C vitamins
- Osteoporosis and anemia
- Diarrhea
- Increased blood pressure and hypertension
- Increased cholesterol and triglyceride blood levels
- Heart rhythm disturbances
- Increased risk of heart attacks (usually in the case of people drinking more than 4 cups a day)
- Fibrostic breast disease
- Birth defects
- Kidney stones
- Increase fevers
- Increased risk of cancers
- Prostate enlargement

- Adrenal fatigue/ hypoglycemia

Caffeine substitutes include
- Roasted Barley
- Chicory Root
- Dandelion Root
- Postum
- Pero
- Pioneer
- Rombouts
- Rostaroma
- Wilson's Heritage
- Cafix
- Miso Broth
- Duran
- Peppermint
- Ginseng Root
- Ginger Root
- Ephedra
- Comfrey Leaf
- Lemon Grass
- Red Clover
- Teccino *

Dietary Supplements and Vitamins

Dietary supplements and vitamin pills do not agree with Islamic medicine because they break the following rules:

They are not natural. They are artificial and man-made. The only exception to this is substances like Barley Green or Fruit Plus where actual whole foods have been dried and enclosed into a bottle in the modern version of preservation.

They cause imbalance in the body because they use the body's resources to be digested and often-times this means that they take minerals, vitamins and nutrients from the body to help in their own absorption. This causes imbalance in the body. The only way this can be avoided is to evaluate each person individually for the exact level of vitamins and minerals they need and then to administer these vitamins and minerals to them according to their daily need. This is being attempted in some circles but still falls a bit short because a person's needs change so frequently that it would be too costly and time-consuming to re-evaluate them as often as needed.

They do have side-effects. There are so many, in fact, that doctors have started to issue warnings *"Don't take vitamin E before surgery (you can bleed to death)"* and other such advice. The following is just one of many examples of how supplements can imbalance the system.

Colloidal Silver

Colloidal silver is a good example of a natural product that is NOT good for you. This is when knowing traditional healing systems in more in depth comes in to play. You cannot blindly consume anything that is "natural" because there is one other important guideline in natural healing – the substance must not cause harm in excess. Some herbs and foods are harmful in excess but they are not toxic. The specific guideline is that the cure must not be toxic. Colloidal silver can be, however.

According to some people, colloidal silver will destroy bacteria in the body and should thus be used as a means to achieving better health. Typically, colloidal silver is created by infusing drinking water with silver ions via an electrical charge. The use of colloidal silver began in the 1800s before the development of antibiotics.

Does colloidal silver destroy bacteria? Actually, silver is used as for legitimate medical purposes in a topical form - silver nitrate, for example, helps treat severe burns. Silver has a long history of being used to retard the growth of bacteria and algae and so have other metals, like copper.

The fact that silver inhibits the growth of living organisms should be the first clue to the fact that it is, on some level, toxic in nature. People who promote its use, however, say that it only affects pathogenic organisms - the nasty things like bacteria, but not human tissue. The truth of the matter is quite different because silver will affect any living cells it comes into contact with. It has no way of knowing that some cells are "good" while others are "bad."

The truth of the matter is also that silver has not been shown to have any positive effects on any of the diseases it is recommended for. On the contrary, the FDA cautions against the use of colloidal silver because the full effects of its toxicity are still unknown. The only sure thing which silver does is cause Argyria. What happens is that, over a long period of time while silver is ingested, the metal is deposited in the skin, organs and other tissues where it remains - a problem which exists with the ingestion of other heavy metals as well. In the end, a person's skin turns a gray or blue-gray color. Permanently.

Cow's Milk

Milk has always been seen as "healthy" so could so many people be wrong? No. Keep in mind that traditionally milk has been:
- Drunk as fresh milk and not pasteurized milk, milk was often most likely from goats and not cows.
- Tradition was also that people would drink what was available in their region so if one was not surrounded by cows it is not logical they should seek cow milk from another region.
- The milk one drinks, according to tradition must be appropriate to the person's constitution (some people should not drink milk at all.)

- The milk on drinks should be fresh and natural (not pasteurized.)
- And the milk one drinks should be in moderation.

Modern medical research, in fact, shows that you are likely to be plagued by anemia, migraine, bloating, gas, indigestion, asthma, prostate cancer, and a host of potentially fatal allergies – especially if you are a person of color. Former Chairman of Pediatrics at Johns Hopkins University, Frank Oski, M.D. even has a book called **Don't Drink Your Milk** which blames every second health problem kids suffer on hormone-ridden commercial milk. Sixty percent of ear infections in kids under six years of age are milk-induced, and milk consumption is the number one cause of iron- deficiency anemia in infants today according to the American Association of Pediatrics. But milk is also a racial issue. Almost 90 percent of African Americans and most Latinos, Asians, and Southern Europeans lack the genes necessary to digest lactose, the primary sugar in milk. Lactose intolerance is the most common "food allergy," but to call it an allergy is to take a white-centric view that trivializes the fact that most of t he world's people are not biologically designed to digest milk.

The late Dr. Benjamin Spock, the U.S.'s leading authority on child care, spoke out against feeding "cow's glue" to children, saying it can cause anemia, allergies, and diabetes and in the long term, will set kids up for obesity and heart disease, the number one cause of death in this country. Most of cow milk's much-vaunted protein is contained in casein – which is also a raw material for commercial glue. Undigested, it simply sticks to the intestinal walls and blocks nutrient absorption.

The controversial Bovine Growth Hormone (BGH) – banned in most countries – is pumped into U.S.A milk cows to increase annual yield (50,000 pounds of milk per cow today compared to 2,000 pounds in 1959). Milk from cows treated with BGH is likely to contain pus from their udders since the hormone leads to mastitis, or udder infection. BGH use results in a tumor-promoting chemical (IGF- I) that has been implicated in an explosive increase of cancer of the colon, smooth muscle, and breast. The antibiotics dairy farmers use around the world to treat BGH-caused infections in cows appear in their milk and greatly hasten human tolerance to most antibiotics, a potentially life- threatening state of affairs. The Center for Science in the Public Interest reports that 38 percent of milk samples in 10 cities were contaminated with sulfa drugs and other antibiotics.

Soda Pop

Soda pop, according to tradition, would not be a healthy substance to drink as it is not natural, but rather is manmade.

However, in today's modern society – here are the statistics: *Carbonated soda pop provides more added sugar in a typical 2-year-old toddler's diet than cookies, candies and ice cream combined. Fifty-six percent of 8-year-olds down soft drinks daily, and a third of teenage boys drink at least three cans of soda pop per day.*

Many adults are part of these statistics as well. And these sodas are even being sold in about 60% of the middle schools nationwide. In countries like Egypt and Saudi Arabia they are sold on every street corner and children drink them as if they were water. In many American schools soda pop vending machines are found (update: in 2005 parents started fighting this with full force and had some success) However, people, including children who are drinking these beverages need to be warned first of the problems they can cause:

Obesity is one problem caused by sodas. Just eliminating sodas in some people's diets can help them lose weight within days. This is because sodas not only contain a lot of sugar, but they also block the absorption of nutrients and enzymes, which help people, digest food. Additionally, sodas with sugar have the added problem of the obesity caused by high sugar consumption. Researchers found that school-children who drank soft drinks consumed almost 200 more calories per day than their counterparts who didn't down soft drinks. That finding helps support the notion that we don't compensate well for calories in liquid form. "Diet" sodas are no better. Read my comments on sweeteners below.

Tooth decay is another problem caused by sodas. A federally funded study of nearly 3,200 Americans 9 to 29 years old conducted between 1971 and 1974 showed a direct link between tooth decay and soft drinks. Numerous other studies have shown the same link throughout the world, from Sweden to Iraq. But sugar isn't the only ingredient in soft drinks that causes tooth problems. The acids in soda pop are also notorious for etching tooth enamel in ways that can lead to cavities. "Acid begins to dissolve tooth enamel in only 20 minutes," notes the Ohio Dental Association.

Caffeine dependence is another problem cause by soda consumption. You can read more about caffeine in the article below. However, did you know that diet sodas contain more caffeine than regular sodas? Labels are not required to contain this information but the facts state this. Regular Coke, for instance has 35 milligrams of caffeine per can. But Diet coke has 42 milligrams in the same size can. A can of Pepsi One has a whopping 56 milligrams. Actually, colas have more powerful effects than many over-the-counter drugs! Furthermore, when you are dependent on a drug, you are really upsetting the normal balances of neurochemistry in the brain. The fact that kids have withdrawal signs and symptoms when the caffeine is stopped is a good indication that something has been profoundly disturbed in the brain.

Another worrisome side effect of sodas is bone weakening. Animal studies demonstrate that phosphorus, a common ingredient in soda, can deplete bones of calcium. And two recent human studies suggest that girls who drink more soda are more prone to broken bones. The industry denies that soda plays a role in bone weakening. Phosphorus -- which occurs naturally in some foods and is used as an additive in many others -- appears to weaken bones by promoting the loss of calcium. With less calcium available, the bones become more porous and prone to fracture. Ironically, going back to the article above (about cow's milk) pasteurized cow's milk actually has increased phosphorus content, which then cancels out some of the benefits of the calcium in the milk.

Last, but not least, the alkaline and acidic levels of the body are thrown off balance by sodas. Scientists have found that healthy people have body fluids that are slightly alkaline, 7.1 to 7.5 pH. Scientists and doctors have also found that over 150degenerative diseases are linked to acidity, including cancer, diabetes, arthritis, heart disease, gall and kidney stones, and many more. All diseases thrive in an acidic, oxygen poor environment. Keep in mind that a drop in every point on the pH scale is10x more acidic than the previous number--i.e. from 7 to 6 is 10x, from 7 to 5 is 100x etc. From 7 to 2 is 100,000x more acidic, colas are in the approximate 2.5 pH range. Almost no soda is higher than 3.0. Diet sodas are the worst as they are highest in acid content. Actually diet sodas can cause you to gain weight because they alter the blood chemistry, making changes in your metabolism, leading to a slower metabolic rate. See my article on Aspartame. The best liquid to drink is water.

Finally, one reason that sodas are so bad, is that soda, like water and some other liquids, pass very quickly through the stomach into the small intestine where it is quickly assimilated into the bloodstream through the openings in the villi in the walls of the intestines. Liquids do not stay in the digestive tract. Almost all liquids go into the bloodstream and is filtered through the liver and the kidneys and whatever is not needed by the body is sent to the bladder and urinated out. But these liquids can come in contact with virtually every cell in your body. When a substance is an acid, it means that there are a large number of positively charged hydrogen ions in the liquid. These positively charged ions are lacking electrons and steal electrons from other atoms in the body which themselves become electrically unstable and seek other electrons from other atoms. These are called free radicals and what you've just started is a chain reaction of electron stealing. The problem with this is that whenever an electron is torn from an atom a little spark is produced, and this known to damage cell membranes. This is called free radical damage and can be seen under a microscope in a live blood cell analysis. The body must stop the process because you would probably die if your body couldn't neutralize the acids. When you use up the supply of available minerals to neutralize the acids, at that point you may get a very serious degenerative disease. Every soda that you drink will contribute to this acidity. Even without soda our bodies naturally produce acids, and minerals are needed in our diets to stop the deterioration process. Unfortunately, most of the food that we eat no longer contains the minerals that we need. This may be the reason for all the degenerative diseases that are so prevalent today.

Sodium Laurel Sulfate & Other Chemicals

Once again the decision whether to use or consume some items comes down to if it is natural or not. Herbal healing tradition makes it clear that people should not consume or use things that are not from nature. Our job is to find a solution in nature and to create "new" solutions in cooperation with nature.

If one consumes or uses manmade chemicals they enter the cycle of the manmade world and sometimes there are no easy solutions then left in nature. Once you enter the realm of the man made you are more and more bound by it, whatever it brings. So as a basic precept of health it is recommended that people stay in the realm of nature. In this realm we are guaranteed solutions for our problems. In the manmade realm, however, there is no guarantee. Oftentimes man will create a product and only come up with a solution for the side-effects ten years later. Often times the side effects do not show up for years to come and sometimes, once the side effects are realized man wishes he never created it to begin with but then it is too late.

Between 1965 and 1982 over 4,000,000 new chemical compounds were formulated. Since then some 6,000 new chemicals have been formulated *weekly*. Approximately 3,000 of these have been formulated to deliberately add to our food. American drinking water contains over 700 chemicals. 884 neuro-toxic chemicals are used in the cosmetic, perfume, and toiletries industries.

One of these chemicals is Sodium Laurel Sulfate, which is also known by some 90 synonyms (such as Product no. 161, or Gardenol) and is used in many products. In America, Warrant Material Safety Data Sheets are available by law. They say of Sodium Laurel Sulfate: "In case of contact, immediately flush the eyes or skin with copious amounts of water for at least 15 minutes while removing contaminated clothing and shoes. Ensure adequate flushing of the eyes by separating the eyelids with the fingers. If inhaled, remove to fresh air. If not breathing, give artificial respiration. If breathing is difficult, give oxygen. If swallowed, wash out the mouth with water. Provided the person is still conscious, call a doctor. When handled, wear approved respirator, chemical-resistant gloves, safety goggles, and other protective clothing. Use only in a chemical fume-hood. Avoid prolonged or repeated exposure. Wash thoroughly after handling. Harmful if inhaled or swallowed. Harmful if absorbed through the skin. Causes severe eye irritation. Causes skin irritation. Materials irritating the mucous membrane upper respiratory tract. Symptoms of exposure may include burning sensation, coughing, wheezing, laryngitis, shortness of breath, headache, nausea, vomiting. May cause allergic respiratory reaction. Significant symptoms of exposure can persist for more than two years. Causes long-term damage to the lungs." Its main industrial use is as an ingredient in floor de- waxers, engine degreasers, garage floor cleaners, and agent orange. Its chief non-industrial use is as a controlled skin irritant in laboratory tests. This is from a news story in the *Daily Mail* 31/7/2001: "Dermatologists ... used seawater to treat cases of dermatitis ... which they induced by treating the skin with sodium lauryl sulfate". Still want it on your skin? So it may surprise you to find out that this is one of the main ingredients in household personal care products. In America, many toothpastes carry a warning label by law because they contain sodium laurel sulfate: "Warning. Keep out of reach of children under 6 years of age. In case of accidental ingestion seek professional assistance or contact a poison control center immediately."

Tobacco

Nicotine elevates the heart rate, which increases the heart's demand for oxygen. At the same time the carbon monoxide in the cigarette reduces the blood's oxygen carrying capacity. The heart is then forced to work with less oxygen. At the same time smoking constricts the arteries, even further restricting the blood supply to the oxygen-impoverished heart. Cigarette smoke also creates a lot of free radicals in the body, which are basically the body's equivalent of "rust." This "rusting" of a person is normal when a person is exposed to a normal life. However, increasing the production of free radicals in the body with cigarettes or air pollution or junk food is akin to continuously washing a tin cup or leaving your bike in the rain. It will quickly rust and fall apart under such abuse.

Tobacco smoke contains more than 4000 chemicals In fact, smoking has been around for centuries, but only since it entered the mainstream of mass production has the bad effects from it skyrocketed. This is because, while moderate smoking of some herbs and grasses may actually be beneficial (This is common in the Native American tradition for example), what you are consuming now in today's modern society is actually a combination of lethal gases (carbon monoxide, hydrogen cyanide, and nitrogen and sulfur oxides) and tars which contain up to 4000 chemicals introduced specially IN the process of making manufactured cigarettes! Cigarettes also contain a high level of polonium which is a strong source of radiation. In fact smoking more than 1 and a half packs per day is equal to getting 300 chest X-rays a year. Smoking is like spraying a sponge with nail polish. The sponge will not then be able to absorb water. The lungs cannot absorb the oxygen it is getting. Oxygen purifies your blood so your blood is carrying more toxins than it should. Each cigarette burns up 25mg of vitamin C. Smokers also need more sulfur as the smoking burns this up as well. Smoking is a known cause in the alternative medicine field of a hiatal hernia. This is because it causes allergic reactions and "explosions" in the stomach involving the hiatal valve. Here are some more things that smoking does:
- Lowers levels of HDL (good) cholesterol.
- Elevates blood pressure by decreasing circulation to peripheral blood vessels
- Destroys lung tissue and invites respiratory infections
- Reduces lung capacity
- Lowers sperm counts in men and reproductive ability
- Reduces the taste for food. Food becomes tasteless.
- Increases risk of hernia, heartburn and peptic ulcers
- *Decreases calcium absorption*

PH (potential of hydrogen) is a measure of the acidity or alkalinity of a solution. It is measured on a scale of 0 to 14—the lower the pH the more acidic the solution, the higher the pH the more alkaline (or base) the solution. When a solution is neither acid nor alkaline it has a pH of 7 which is neutral. The alchemists would have loved playing with this concept!

Water is the most abundant compound in the human body, comprising 70% of the body. The body has an acid-alkaline (or acid-base) ratio called the pH which is a balance between positively charges ions (acid-forming) and negatively charged ions (alkaline-forming.) The body continually strives to balance pH. When this balance is compromised many problems can occur.

It is important to understand that we are not talking about stomach acid or the pH of the stomach. We are talking about the pH of the body's fluids and tissues which is an entirely different matter. Most people who suffer from unbalanced pH are acidic. This condition forces the body to borrow minerals—including calcium, sodium, potassium and magnesium—from vital organs and bones to buffer (neutralize) the acid and safely remove it from the Most people who suffer from unbalanced pH are acidic. This condition forces the body to borrow minerals—including calcium, sodium, potassium and magnesium—from vital organs and bones to buffer (neutralize) the acid and safely remove it from the body. Because of this strain, the body can suffer severe and prolonged damage due to high acidity—a condition that may go undetected for years.

Mild acidosis can cause such problems as:
- Cardiovascular damage, including the constriction of blood vessels and the reduction of oxygen.
- Weight gain, obesity and diabetes.
- Bladder and kidney conditions, including kidney stones.
- Immune deficiency.
- Acceleration of free radical damage, possibly contributing to cancerous mutations.
- Premature aging.
- Osteoporosis; weak, brittle bones, hip fractures and bone spurs.
- Joint pain, aching muscles and lactic acid buildup.

The reason acidosis is more common in our society is mostly due to the typical American diet, which is far too high in acid-producing animal products like meat, eggs and dairy, and far too low in alkaline-producing foods like fresh vegetables. Additionally, we eat acid-producing processed foods like white flour and sugar and drink acid-producing beverages like coffee and soft drinks. We use too many drugs, which are acid-forming; and we use artificial chemical sweeteners like NutraSweet, Equal, or aspartame, which are extremely acid-forming. One of the best things we can do to correct an overly-acid body is to clean up the diet and lifestyle. Refer to the recommended reading for specific help with diet and lifestyle.

General Food Categories to be aware of when following your "normal" diet.

Categories	Lowest Alkaline	Lowest Acid	Acid	Most Acid
Dairy	Soy Cheese, Soy Milk, Goat Milk, Goat Cheese, Whey	Eggs, Butter, Yogurt, Buttermilk, Cottage Cheese	Raw Milk	Cheese, Homogenized Milk, Ice Cream
Drinks	Ginger Tea	Tea	Coffee	Beer, Soft Drinks
Fruits	Oranges, Bananas, Cherries, Pineapple, Peaches, Avocados	Plums, Processed Fruit Juices	Sour Cherries, Rhubarb	Blueberries, Cranberries, Prunes
Grains	Amaranth, Millet, Wild Rice, Quinoa	Sprouted Wheat Bread, Spelt, Brown Rice	White Rice, Corn, Buckwheat, Oats, Rye	Wheat, White Flour, Pastries, Pasta
Meats		Venison, Cold Water Fish	Turkey, Chicken, Lamb	Beef, Pork, Shellfish
Nuts	Chestnuts	Pumpkin Seeds, Sunflower Seeds	Pecans, Cashews	Peanuts, Walnuts
Oils	Canola Oil	Corn Oil		
Sweets	Raw Honey, Raw Sugar	Processed Honey, Molasses	White Sugar, Brown Sugar	NutraSweet, Equal, Aspartame, Sweet 'N Low
Vegetables	Carrots, Tomatoes, Fresh Corn, Mushrooms, Cabbage, Peas, Potato Skins, Olives, Soybeans, Tofu	Cooked Spinach, Kidney Beans, String Beans	Potatoes (without skins), Pinto Beans, Navy Beans, Lima Beans	Chocolate

Note that a food's acid or alkaline-forming tendency in the body has nothing to do with the actual pH of the food itself. For example, lemons are very acidic, however the end-products they produce after digestion and assimilation are very alkaline so lemons are alkaline-forming in the body. Likewise, meat will test alkaline before digestion but it leaves very acidic residue in the body so, like nearly all animal products, meat is very acid-forming. The following is a diet that I have my clients follow to help them re-balance. It is a good diet to do for ten days now and then to make sure you are in balance. Some people, in fact, make a habit of eating like this. One thing I like about this diet is it teaches people moderation in eating.

Studies of Dietary Supplements Come Under Growing Scrutiny

Excerpt By Ford Fessenden,The New York Times

When a California judge handed down a $12.5 million false-advertising judgment against the maker of an ephedra-based weight-loss pill late last month, he also issued what amounted to a bill of reproach against the science of dietary supplements. The company, Cytodyne Technologies, maker of Xenadrine RFA-1, the supplement implicated in the death of a Baltimore Orioles pitcher, had not just exaggerated the findings of clinical trials it commissioned, Superior Court Judge Ronald L. Styn said in ruling on a class-action suit, but had also cajoled some researchers into fudging results in published Scientific articles. This is raising serious questions about the way makers of ephedra and other dietary supplements use - and often misuse - the promise of scientific proof to market their products. In the last eight months, three leading manufacturers of weight-loss pills have been hit with false-advertising verdicts in the millions of dollars. A fourth has been rebuked by a federal judge for hiding evidence. The Missouri attorney general and a group of district attorneys in California have also brought false-advertising suits against manufacturers, and Congress has demanded Cytodyne's research records.

Assignment for Section Two

There are many foods and chemicals we put into our bodies that are harmful. In Chapter 2 I explore some of these items. Please explain, in your OWN WORDS, and using only three sentences at the most, one or two reasons why the following items could be harmful Please write two-four paragraphs on one ADDITIONAL item that is NOT included on the list above. Topics you could use include: recreational drugs, artificial colorings, artificial flavorings, prescription drugs, over-the-counter drugs, sugar, excess meat, anything you can think of that fits into this category.

~Section Three: The Four Humors and Nutrition~

The History and Theory of Temperament in Islamic Medicine
by Kristie Karima Burns, Mh, ND

This article shows how the temperaments were viewed by Islamic Medicine. This view was/is shared by many other cultures and experts. "The Four Humors" is a classic way to view the body in traditional healing all around the world. In fact, "typing" people is so popular it is even used in modern times during job interviews.

"Lo! In the creation of the heavens and the earth, and the difference of night and day, and the ships which run upon the sea with that which is of use to men, and the water which Allah sendeth down from the sky; thereby reviving the earth after its death, and dispersing all kinds of beasts therein, and (in) the ordinance of the winds, and the clouds obedient between heaven and earth: are signs (of Allah's sovereignty) for people who have sense" (Sura'tul Baqarah, 2:164).

According to Avicenna, Allah made all kinds of people as well as all kinds of beasts and they can be roughly categorized into four types. In fact, as far back as Hippocrates in 450 BC, the idea that people could be categorized according to "types" was very popular and was used as a key to self- development, relationships, job choice, and even health care and maintenance. Hippocrates, and later Avicenna, defined these types as sanguine, choleric, melancholic, and phlegmatic and taught how each type could live a healthier and more personally rewarding life. As Muslims, we can use this insight to help our community grow together, to nurture family relationships, to inspire self- improvement and to heal ourselves.

Physically, the sanguine element has historically represented the nutritive aspect of metabolism; the choleric element, the stimulating and heating aspect; the phlegmatic element, the fluid, cooling and purifying aspects; and the melancholic element, the coagulating, solidifying, drying and concentrating aspects. A quick definition of each temperament personality usually notes its reaction to stimuli in their environment. Thus, the sanguine temperament is marked by quick but shallow, superficial excitability; the choleric is characterized by a quick but strong and lasting reaction; the melancholic temperament is defined by his slow but deep response and the phlegmatic is famous for his slow but shallow excitability. The first two are extroverts and the last two are introverts.In the Qur'an, Allah describes man as being created from water *(32:8)*, *"which is cold and wet; earth" (3:59)*, *"which is cold and dry; clay"* (7:12), *"which is cold and wet; and a sounding clay" (55:14)*, *"which is hot and wet as it is transformed or hot and dry as it is beaten by the wind."*

Although the terms used in the Qur'an vary from the terms used by temperamental "healers" during the time of Prophet Muhammad (SAW), the elemental qualities of man remain consistent. Thus, the sanguine element corresponds to the hot and wet sounding clay as it is transformed; the choleric element corresponds to the hot and dry sounding clay as it is beaten by the wind; the melancholic element corresponds to the cold and dry earth; and the phlegmatic element corresponds to the cold and wet water (or raw clay). Although Allah was said to have created each person to have all of these elements, practitioners of temperamental healing have observed that each person usually contains a predominate element.

The opposing idea that all people are alike is a twentieth century idea stemming from the 'democratic' idea that if we are all going to be free and equal that we must also be alike. Many popular books on the modern market propel this idea even farther. Books like 'The McDougall Plan', 'The Zone', and 'The Atkin's Diet' all claim that their diets are the best for everyone and largely discredit any claims that different diets may benefit different types. Furthermore, most discipline books recommend raising children using only one form of discipline and most self-help books recommend that their method is the "one and only" way to success. On the other hand, books like 'Eat Right 4 Your Type', 'Between Heaven and Earth' (a book on Chinese Healing) and 'The Medicine of The Prophet' each emphasize the importance of recognizing people's health needs according to their various types.

Historically, Islamic society allowed equality but does not define equality with being alike. For example, in the Qur'an it says:(9:71) *"And (as for) the believing men and the believing women, they are guardians of each other; they enjoin good and forbid evil and keep up prayer and pay the poor-rate, and obey Allah and His Apostle; (as for) these, Allah will show mercy to them; surely Allah is Mighty, Wise"(9:72) "Allah has promised to the believing men and the believing women gardens, beneath which rivers flow, to abide in them, and goodly dwellings in gardens of perpetual abode; and best of all is Allah's goodly pleasure; that is the grand achievement"*.

The fallacy of equality through being alike is extremely evident in the women's movement of the 1960's and 1970's that sought to create equality of the sexes by turning women into men. This failed because women and men are unique. They can only be equal if they work to improve their unique qualities within their own functional boundaries. In much the same way, the theory of temperament states that people in general must also function within their own boundaries and type. Rather than struggling to become something they are not, or abusing others because they are not as they expect them to be, people must develop themselves and appreciate others according to the gifts Allah has given them. Many mainstream Americans have difficulty using this valuable system of healing because they cannot get beyond the idea that "everyone must be the same to be equal or right".

Many Christian writers have also explored the temperaments, however, many were largely rejected by the church because some church authorities say that since it is not written in the Bible it cannot be true. Even so, a number of modern Christian writers have gained much popularity in the past ten years for their spiritual insights into the classical temperament system. Some of these writers are even claiming that the system of temperaments is inherently Christian. These writers are: Tim LaHaye, (Spirit-Controlled Temperament (1967); Transformed Temperaments (1971); and Why You Act the Way You Do (1984), Florence Littauer, Charles Stanley, Larry Burkett and John G. MacArthur.

Muslims at the time in history they were emerging were uniquely suited to gain from the scientific research in this field as the prophet Muhammad gave them permission to, *"Seek knowledge from the cradle to the grave... even as far as China"* and also emphasized the uniqueness of the individual within the equality of the society. In other words, Islam had no problem accepting the idea and usefulness of the system of temperaments.

Some of the most prominent Muslim scientists, such as Avicenna explored the theory of temperaments in great detail and an entire field of Islamic Medicine called Unani Tibb, is devoted to healing through the temperaments. Healing through temperaments was popular at the time of the prophet and some of the methods the prophet mentions in the Hadith such as cupping and cautery were popular "balancing" methods in this field of medicine. In addition, the hadiths frequently refer to the 'hot' and 'cold' qualities of foods, which was another tool used by this healing system.

Avicenna developed his theories based on the Hippocratic definition of the four humors which existed in the body called black bile, phlegm, blood and yellow bile. Before Hippocrates, however, the ancient Greeks had at least three humors they worked with which very much resemble the present day Ayurvedic system of temperament and healing. The idea of four humors, though, most likely originated with Hippocrates, who observed upon examining blood that the red portion of fresh blood is the blood humor, the white material mixed with blood is the phlegm, the yellow-colored froth on top is the yellow bile, and the heavy part that settles down is the black bile (sauda).

Avicenna developed this Hippocratic method even farther when he stated that intercellular and extracellular fluids were secondary humors and that the origin and action the four humors or essences (Arabic: akhlat) and their ultimate fate in the digestive process are affected by diet. Avicenna defines the elements as simple substances which provide the primary components of the human body. Although he also recognized the substances of blood, black & yellow bile and phlegm, he also correlated these to the four elements of earth, air, water and fire and assigned these four elements temperamental qualities of cold, hot, moist and dry. He also pointed out that although there is a close association between a body fluid and its humor, the humor is considered separate and independent of the body fluid.

Other Arab Muslim Physicians who used the theories of temperament are Abu Bakr Muhammad Zakariya Al Razi (865AD), Ibn Qayyim Al-Jawziyya (1292), and Jalalu'd-Din Abd'ur-Rahman ibn Bakr as-Suyuti (1445). All speak extensively in their works on the humors and how a practitioner can heal the sick through balancing of the humors.

Plato (340), Aristotle (325) , Adickes (1907), Spranger (1914) , Kretchmer (1920), Fromm (1947), Meyers (1955) and Keirsey (1987) have all explored the four temperaments in their own way as well. Even Winnie The Pooh explored the temperaments using Pooh as an example of the melancholic, Rabbit as the choleric, Tigger as the sanguine and Eeyore as the phlegmatic type.

Islamic Unani Tibb Medicine was formed by refining the theories of Hippocrates, Avicenna and later Arab physicians even farther. Unani Tibb recognizes the four humors, the corresponding elemental qualities and temperamental qualities. However, Unani Tibb further divides the human being into 2 'virtues' and 3 'faculties'. Using the four element system, Unani Tibb recognizes that each human is made up primarily of the progressive and procreative virtue and a second, physiological virtue. They also define people as being divided into corresponding and interactive faculties which are called: the vital faculty which is akin to the spiritual side of a person, the natural faculty which is akin to the physical being of a person and the psychic faculty, which has little to do with "psychic" ability, but actually relates to the conscious and unconscious mind. It is believed that a person is born into a certain temperament though their physical.

The Three Schools of Greek Medicine

by Kristie Karima Burns, Mh, ND

It is evident that among such a group of peoples as the Greeks, varying in state of civilization, in mental power, in geographical and economic position and in general outlook, the practice of medicine can have been by no means uniform. Without any method of centralizing medical education and standardizing teaching there was a great variety of doctrine's and of practice in vogue among them, and much of this was on a low level of folk custom. Back in B.C. Greek civilization there were three different schools of medicine which you could belong, the Cinidian school, the Coan school, and the Alexandrian school of Medicine. Below is a vague outline of the three schools. All of the information is not in this outline yet.

The Cinidian School
- Euryphon was its best known physician and founder of the school. He was skilled in anatomy, wrote much on remedies, and was particularly known for writing on human milk from the breast for consumptives (people who had tuberculosis).
- Their approaches to disease are indebted to the Egyptians.
- Herodias was a gymnastics trainer who turned physician and became famous for over-exercising his patients, even in fever.
- The Cnidians divided up diseases according to symptoms, over-emphasized diagnosis, and over-elaborated treatment.
-

The Coan School
- Draws from Mesopotamian tradition in medicine.
- Best and largest of the three schools.
- Hippocrates is the school's leader.
- Coan physicians took opportunities for gaining experience in anatomy afforded by warfare.

They laid very great force on prognosis and adopted a largely expectant (wait and see) attitude towards diseases.

Empedocles of Agrigentum (c.500-c.430 BC) led to the belief that the heart is the center of the vascular system and the chief organ of the **pneuma** (blood) which was distributed by the blood vessels. This belief was rejected by the Coan school. Anaximenes (c.610-c.545 B.C.), an Ionian predecessor of Empedocles, defined the function of the **pneuma**.

Pythagoras of Samos (c.580-c.490 B.C.) believed that the number was the basis of philosophy. This is his equation: The universe was represented by: 2 and was divided by the number: 12 whence we have three worlds and four spheres. These in turn, according at least to the later Pythagoreans, give rise to the four elements, earth, air, fire, and water---a primary doctrine of medicine and of science derived from ancient Egypt. The following is the thoughts on these four HUMORS, and what they meant to the rest of the Greeks.

The Four Humors

	Water	Air	Fire	Earth
Qualities	Cold and Wet	Hot and Wet	Hot and Dry	Cold and Dry
Humor	Phlegm	Blood	Yellow Bile	Black Bile
Body Part	Brain	Blood	Liver	Spleen

With the rise of Greek Civilization, physical ills in the West were no longer blamed on the gods or sin, but on imbalance within the body itself. The Greeks, like the Indians and the Chinese, believed in balance. To be balanced the Four Humors must not be disturbed. If they were disturbed the result would be disease. "The Greeks believed in the existence of four fluids, or humors, within the body, the balance of which was vital for health. The humors corresponded to the four elements, and had the same qualities; they were also associated with particular parts of the body.

Alexandrian School

Alcmaeon of Croton (c. 500 B.C.) a pupil of Pythagoras. He began to construct a positive basis for medical science by the practice of dissection of animals, and discovered the optic nerve (in your eyes) and the Eustachian tubes. He also studied embryology (the study of the development of a child from the point where sperm meets egg to birth) and described the head as being the first part of the fetus (unborn child) to develop. He also said that health depends on harmony, disease on discord of the elements (earth, air, fire, water...as mentioned above) within the body.

The History of Temperament and Temperament Theory
by Kristie Karima Burns, Mh, ND

"Tradition has it that fat men are jolly and generous, that lean men are dour, that short men are aggressive, and that strong men are silent and confident. But tradition is sometimes wise and sometimes stupid, for seldom does it distinguish between the accumulated wisdom of the ages and the superstitions of ignorance."

The doctrine of temperament can be traced to the theory of humors which is a microcosmic form of the macrocosmic theory of the four elements (earth, water, air, fire) as first proposed by Empedocles (V B.C.) and the four qualities (dry, wet, cold, hot). Humoral theory states that there are four body humors, and their proper mixture is the condition of health. The theory is ascribed to the school of *Cos* and more precisely to Polybos, son-in- law to Hippocrates (Sarton, 1954). Before him, the greek hylozoists had devoted their attention to the cause of illness and the function of the humors as evidenced in the teachings of Anaxagoras and more so in those of Democratis and Alcmeon (Roback, 1928).

The four humors are fluid substances: blood, phlegm, yellow bile, and black bile. A healthy condition is a result of balanced proportions to each of the humors in respect to their combination, strength, and quality. Discomfort and pain result from either a deficiency or excess of any one or combination of these fluids. Each humor/fluid is differentiated by its color, evident tactile differences, degree of warmth or cold, and differences in dryness and moisture making temperaments subject to seasonal and temperate influence. The principles of therapy were based on cure by opposites (allopathy) (Levine, 1971).

The theory of temperaments was the fourth in this dialectic ascension of theories. Temperament theory suggested that though the proportions of the humors may vary considerably, they could be reduced to four types of mixtures or temperaments (crasis) according to the predominance of a given humor. Since there were four humors, it was proposed that there could only be four temperaments and therefore four kinds of healthy equilibrium, not one, and that men could be subdivided into four psychological groups named after the prevalent humor: the sanguine, buoyant type; the phlegmatic, sluggish type; the choleric, quick-tempered type; and the melancholic, dejected type. The theory was alluded to in the Hippocratic The Nature of Man (Peri physios anthropou) and its elaboration was continued by Eristratos (III-1B.C.) and by Asclepiades (I-1B.C.). The Greek physician Galen's (130-200A.D.) treatise, Pericraison, De temperamentis was so well formulated that it remained the standard authority until the 16th century, when Andreas Vesalius and, later, William Harvey amended Galen's theories with their medical discoveries.

East Indian traditional Ayurvedic medicine has its basis in humoral theories. That is, the human body is a macrocosm of the universe. The seven body substances-bone, flesh, fat, blood, semen, marrow, and chyle-are the product of three humors: kapha, or phlegm; pitta, or bile; and vata, or wind. Health depends on the equilibrium of these humors, and sickness is a disequilibrium. The point of equilibrium depends on age, sex, temperament, climate, nutrition, and the nature of daily activities. A smaller branch of traditional medicine on the subcontinent, and one common to Muslim areas, is the practice of Yunani or Unani. This is the medicine of the ancient Greeks, translated into Arabic and Persian and then slowly modified by its practitioners, the Hakim. The works of Galen are accepted figuratively and in detail. True to this Mediterranean tradition, the medicine has four humors: yellow bile, black bile, phlegm, and blood. These humors combine with the four primary qualities of heat, cold, moisture, and dryness. If the humors and qualities are in equilibrium, a person is healthy; if not, illness results.

Human differences have been the subject of faith, theory, and observance throughout history. Gnosticism was a religious philosophical dualism that professed salvation through secret knowledge, or gnosis. The movement reached a high point of development during the 2nd century A.D. in the Roman and Alexandrian schools founded by Valentius. The Gnostic sects set forth their teachings in complex systems of thought. Characteristic of their position was the doctrine that all material reality was evil. Central to their convictions of salvation is the freeing of the spirit from its imprisonment in matter. In Gnostic thought, a divine seed is imprisoned in every person. The purpose of salvation is to deliver this lost seed.

Gnostics classified people according to these three categories. (1) Gnostics, or those certain of salvation, because they were under the influence of the spirit (pneumatikoi); (2) those not fully Gnostic, but capable of salvation through knowledge (psychikoi); and (3) those so dominated by mater that they were beyond salvation (hylikoi). Temperament theory played a predominant role in Gnostic faith.

Wycliff's sermons, published in 1380, appear to be among the first English literature to allude to the temperaments, or rather, the humors. Shakespeare described the four temperaments in Cynthia's Revels and later in Every Man Out of His Humor. Robert Burton's Anatomy of Melancholy provides a detailed description of the humoral doctrine. Further speculations arrived with the onset of the scientific revolutions of Copernicus, Galilei, and Harvey. At the onset of the eighteenth century, Andreas Rudiger in his Physica Divina reduced the number of elements responsible for temperamental differences to two: *aither* as cause of the light qualities, and *air* as cause of the heavy qualities. With Harvey's discoveries of the circulation of the blood, temperament emphasis shifted from the composition of the blood to its movement as the determinant of differences in temperament. *"In a word, the humoral doctrine was beginning to change into a solid theory."* (Roback, 1928, p.48).

Stahl and later Hoffman, proposed to take into consideration three factors into their temperament theory: (a) the constitution of the blood, (b) the porosity of the tissue, and (c) the width of the blood vessels. Haller in the middle of the eighteenth century laid the beginnings of modern experimental physiology resulting in the theory of humors receiving a permanent setback. Haller proposed that the connection between the blood and the temperaments is not a necessary one but that parts through which the blood flows, or rather their strength and irritability, are fundamental in accounting for temperamental differences. With research in nerve physiology, the doctrine of temperaments took a new direction. The nervous system was not to be the seat of temperament (Roback, 1928). Chief among the new scholars was a student of Haller. Wrisberg combined the four humors into a double category: choleric-sanguine, and melancholic-phlegmatic.

At this same time, the science of philosophy stepped in to *"dismiss all the materialistic theories as either worthless or so highly speculative as to be of little assistance"* (Roback, 1928, p.50). Plater's Philosophische Aphorismen and Kant's Anthropolgie produced new sets of temperaments. Platter proposed that temperaments be composed of: (a) the attic or mental, derived from the preponderance of the higher physic organ (auditory, visual, and tactile); (b) the animal temperament, resulting from the preponderance of the second organ over the first; (c) the heroic temperament, where both organs or systems are well matched; and (d) the faint temperament produced by the lack of energy in either of the two organs. Kant's treatment of character places temperament between two marks of individuality which he calls *characteristic* and *character*. Temperament is regarded by Kant to be a mode of sensibility. *"The temperaments he considers both as physiological facts, such as physical constitution and complexion of humors, and psychological tendencies due to the composition of the blood"* (Roback, 1928, p.52).

The phrenologistic teachings of Gall and Spurtzheim attempted to create a new science which purported to localize abilities and disabilities to specific regions of the brain, and dismissing the determinate faculties. Spurtzheim in *Phrenology in Connection with the Study of Physiognomy* considered the study of temperaments as the first step in phrenology. Phrenological temperaments became known as (a) the motive, based on the muscular system, (b) the vital, indicating a predominance of the alimentary system, and (c) the mental temperament, drawing its strength from the nervous system.

Toward the middle of the eighteenth century, the French physician Halle distinguished between general temperaments, partial temperaments, and acquired temperaments. General temperaments were linked with the vascular, nervous, and motor systems. Partial temperaments corresponded to the various regions of the body and the fluids, pituita, and bile. The acquired temperaments resulted from environmental influences on the primary temperaments (Roback, 1928).

The study of temperament in the nineteenth century represents an embodiment of ideas from immediate predecessors. Influenced by the powers of electricity, Schelling felt that temperaments shared the same fate of opposites as did electricity. Organisms were said to contain two polar principles of gravity and light (substance and movement) which *"were it not for the predominance of the one or the other in the individual, would yield total identity, where all differences would be obliterated"* (Roback, 1928, p.63). Temperament anomalies occurred when there was an imbalance in the three dimensions. Temperaments according to Johannes Muller became the forms of psychic life. A co-worker of Muller, the German-Jewish anatomist Jacob Henle, based his theory of temperaments on the tone of the nervous system, speed of the reaction and its duration (Roback, 1928).

In 1795, Shiller conceptualized two psychological types, the *Idealist* and the *Realist*. The German philosopher Friedrich Wilhelm Nietzsche in his first book, <u>The Birth of Tragedy</u> (1872; English translation, 1968), introduced his famous distinction between the Appolonian, or rational, element in human nature and the Dionysian, or passionate, element as exemplified in the Greek gods Apollo and Dionysis. With a blend of the two principles, either in art or in life, humanity achieves a momentary harmony with the Primordial Mystery. The Swiss writer of epic poetry, stories, novels, dramas, and essays, Carl Georg Friedrich Spittler in his epic *Prometheus and Epimetheus* (1881; English translation, 1931), reflecting the pessimism of Schopenhauer and the romantacism of Niezsche describes two types called *Prometheus* and *Epimetheus*.

In 1892, Pilo's <u>Nuovi Studi sul Caratter</u> looked for the basic differences of man in the chemical composition of the blood and its thermicity. Pilo identifies four general temperament characters: the plethoric, the serious, the bilious, and the lymphatic. In 1907, Dr. Erich Adickes proposed dividing man into four world views: dogmatic, agnostic, traditional, and innovative. Alfred Adler spoke similarly of four mistaken goals: recognition, power, service, and revenge. In 1920, Eduard Spranger told of four human values that set people apart: religious, theoretic, economic, and artistic (Keirsey, 1984). The American philosopher and psychologist

William James, one of the founders and leading proponents of pragmatism, considered philosophies to be expressions of personal temperament and developed a correlation between *tough-minded* and *tender-minded* temperaments and empiricist and rationalist positions in philosophy.

Carl Gustav Jung (1923), felt he possessed two separate personalities: an outer public self-involved with the world and his family and peers and a secret inner self that felt a special closeness to God. The interplay between these selves formed a central theme of Jung's personal life and contributed to his later emphasis on the individual's st of four psychological functions or *types* is most highly developed: thinking, feeling, sensation, or intuition.

Shortly after the publication of Jung's book, <u>Psychological Types</u>, Ernst Kretschmerriving for integration and wholeness. Jung proposed that motivation be understood in terms of a general creative life energy-the libido-capable of being invested in different directions and assuming a variety of different forms. The two principal directions of the libido are extroversion (outward into the world of other people and objects) and introversion (inward into the realm of images, ideas, and the unconscious). Persons in whom the former directional tendency predominates are extroverts, while those in whom the latter is strongest are introverts. Jung also proposed to group people according to which (1925) published his book, <u>Physique and Character</u> in which he describes the *"Cycloid"* and *"Schizoid"* types. In 1942, William Sheldon published <u>The Varieties of Temperament</u> in which he presents a system for treating the problem of individual differences in terms of what appears to be basic components of temperament. These components in turn are tied back to and interpreted in terms of basic components of morphology. The emphasis is upon the constitutional factors, upon the relatively stable qualities of an individual that give him his basic individuality. Sheldon's study extended through a period of five years analyzing the morphological and temperamental characteristics of 200 young men. Sheldon created a scale for temperament based upon 60 traits categorized into three groups: Viscerotonia-characterized by general relaxation, love of comfort,sociability, congeniality, gluttony for food, for people, and for affection; Somatotonia-characterized by a predominance of muscular activity and of vigorous bodily assertiveness; and Cerbratotonia-characterized by a predominance of the element of restraint, inhibition, and of the desire for concealment.

A major breakthrough in *typology* came in 1942 with the emergence of the *Myers Briggs Type Indicator* (MBTI). Isabelle Myers and Katherine Briggs based their conceptual framework on the typology created by Carl Jung. They felt that differences concern the way people prefer to use their minds, specifically the way in which people make judgements. Myers and Briggs identified *"perceiving"* as the process of becoming aware of things, people, occurrences, and ideas. *"Judging"* includes the perceived process of coming to conclusions. Together, perception and judgement govern much of one's outer behavior.

Joseph Hill (NP) looked to develop in education the level of precision and accountability found in medicine and law. He based his work on Gestalt psychology and research by Kagan and Witkin. Hill developed the concept of cognitive style mapping and the classification of learners in terms of sensory preference; Auditory, Visual, or Tactile-Kinesthetic.

In 1928, *William Marston* in EmotionsofNormalPeople investigated motor consciousness as the basis of feeling and emotion. Marston's psychonic theory of consciousness traced the affective consciousness to mechanistic-type causes; that is, to nerve impulses, thence to bodily changes and, ultimately, to environmental stimuli. Marston viewed people as having two axis with their actions tending to be active or passive depending upon the individual's perception of the environment as either antagonistic or favorable. By placing these axis at right angles, four quadrants were formed with each circumscribing a behavior pattern; dominance produces activity in an antagonistic environment, inducement produces activity in a favorable environment, steadiness produces passivity in a favorable environment, and compliance produces passivity in an antagonistic environment. Marston proposed that learning by inducement and submission is pleasant; learning by trial and error (compliance and dominance) is painful.

Walter Clark's Activity Vector Analysis (AVA) was developed as a psychometric instrument around Marston's theory. John Geier's (1972) PersonalProfile:WORKBehaviorCharacteristic Interpretation, describes behaviors in terms of how others see you, your behavior under pressure, and how you see yourself. This theory of dimensional behavior adheres to the precept that behavior changes can and does take place. The four-section indicator developed by Geier tests for Dominance (D), Influence (I), Steadiness (S), and Compliance (C).

Keith Golay, 1982) described four basic and distinct learning types by the individual's pattern of learning. Based on the work of David Keirsey and Marilyn Bates, as well as Isabelle Myers, Golay believes that personality predisposes the learner to certain ways of thinking, wanting, liking, and acting. Golay classifies learners as; Actual Spontaneous, Actual Routine, Conceptual Specific, or Conceptual Global.

David Keirsey (1984) combined Kretschmer's temperament hypothesis with Jung's behavior description, and with Nietzsche's and Spitteler's Greek typology. Keirsey notes themes in the various observations and the consistent tendency of human behavior. He observed four patterns: Sensing Perceiver (SP), Sensing Judger (SJ), Intuitive Thinker (NT), and Intuitive Feeler (NF). These four patterns are temperaments-the way in which human personality interacts with the environment.

The Physical Characteristics of Temperament

by Kristie Karima Burns, Mh, ND

Traditional, classical, and modern experts in all religions and healing systems agree that a person is born with a predominance of one element over the others (determining their temperament). They refer to these different elements as sanguine (hot and wet), choleric (hot and dry), melancholic (cold and dry), and phlegmatic (cold and wet). Many traditional healers in the area of Unani Tibb, Ayurveda and Chinese Medicine as well as Classical Western Herbalism, teach that healing is merely a matter of balancing these elements (or humors) in a person through physical, emotional and spiritual channels.

This article will discuss each of the temperaments, their manifestation in the body, and the best manner for a person with that predominate temperament (either naturally or temporarily) to achieve general good health and/or healing. Each humor has a corresponding personality profile; these will be outlined in Part Two of this series.

Samuel Hahnemann, the father of homeopathy, recognized the importance of knowing a person's temperament in determining how they would be affected by disease and how they would react to different medicines. In his essay, "Suppression in the Four Hippocratic Temperaments," he observed that each type reacted differently to the medical suppression of rashes. Sanguine people suffer piles, hemorrhoids, colic, and renal gravel after the suppression of an itch whereas phlegmatic people suffer from dropsy and delayed menses after such suppression. Melancholic people become mentally imbalanced or sterile.

Hahnemann stated, "Each innate constitutional temperament has its own unique reactions to stimuli. For this reason, the same pathogen will affect the four temperaments and their 12 mixtures in a different manner. For example, the phlegmatic and melancholic temperaments are usually aggravated by cold, while the choleric and sanguine temperament are usually ameliorated by cold." The sanguine element, as a physiological trait, stimulates the veins and arteries and provides the motivational energy of the body. Signs of excess sanguine humor are usually displayed in a person's circulatory system - their veins are bigger (or at least appear so) and fuller than ordinary; their skin is red or reddens easily; they may have pricking pains in their sides and about their temples; they may sometimes experience shortness of breath or headache; and may have thick, colored urine. Practitioners have observed over time that many "sanguines" possess all or some of the following qualities: ruddy, smooth, firm, moist and warm skin; dark brown or fair hair; hairy body; medium stature; muscular body build; a good appetite; quick and good digestion; light yellow urine; firm brown feces; happy dreams and a general happy nature.

Sanguine types are often light-footed and rhythmical much like their counterpart, the circulatory system. They usually have expressive faces and "sparkling eyes," and may often have curly or wavy, rather than straight, hair. The sanguine will be most extreme or imbalanced during the spring or summer, or when exposed to wind or heat (while going out in the heat to shop or from leaving the car window open while driving, etc.), and after eating sour, greasy, and spicy foods.

Physiologically, the choleric element is closely associated with the nervous system, acting to increase the rate at which it functions. It has a warming effect on the body, stimulates the intellect, and increases physical and mental activity and courage. Its receptacle is the gall bladder. Signs of excess choleric humor are: leanness of body; hollow eyes; anger without a cause; a testy disposition; yellowness of the skin; bitterness in the throat; pricking pains in the head; a swifter and stronger pulse than typical; troublesome sleeps; and dreams of fire, lightning, anger and/or fighting. Practitioners have also observed that choleric persons also possess many of the following qualities: yellow, rough, warm and dry skin; dark brown or red hair; very hairy bodies; short stature; a lean body build; a strong appetite; overactive digestion; thick orange urine; and dry and yellow feces.

The choleric type may experience problems with anxiety, agitation, frenzy, nervous exhaustion, and insomnia. They may also have palpitations, hypoglycemia, rashes, palsy, or strokes. Cholerics tend to incline toward mind-altering substances (anything from coffee to chocolate or alcohol and both prescription and illicit drugs), and they typically have problems with disturbed sleep; bed-wetting as children; heart disturbances; disturbances of speech or sensation; and blood pressure and circulation problems.

In *The Traditional Healer's Handbook*, the melancholic element is described as "consisting of a cool and thick earthly aspect which is prone to coagulation and a more fluid, vaporous substance." In normal quantities, it stimulates memory and creates a homely, practical, pragmatic, and studious nature. However, its coldest part is adherent and, if not eliminated properly, it can settle on or in tissues and form tumors. The spleen, its receptacle, removes the melancholic element from the blood and body fluids. Signs of excess melancholy element are: fearfulness without a cause; a fearful and foolish imagination; rough and swarthy skin; leanness; want of sleep; frightful dreams; sourness in the throat; weak pulse; solitariness; thin clear urine; and frequent sighing. Melancholic types may often display the following characteristics: brown, rough, dry, cold skin; dark brown or black hair; balding hair; medium or slim body build; large appetite; slow digestion; thick, pale urine; dry and black feces; nightmares; and worry or grief.

Melancholics tend to drag their feet and act as if their bodies were a burden to them. They often experience major physical pain from even the most minor injuries. The phlegmatic element, as a physiological trait, functions to expel excess and unnecessary substances from the body. Phlegm plays a necessary role in the body during bouts with the cold and flu; however, copious amounts of it are expelled by the body through the nose in an attempt to clear out toxins and bacteria. The phlegmatic humor has a beneficial cooling and moistening effect on the heart, and strengthens the function of the lower brain and the emotions. Phlegm maintains proper fat metabolism and the balance of body fluids, electrolytes, and hormones through the circulation of lymph and moisture through the body in the same manner that sanguine, or blood, provides nutrition through the circulation system. Its receptacle is the lungs. Signs of excess phlegm in the system can be exhibited by sleepiness; dullness;

slowness; heaviness; cowardliness; forgetfulness; frequent spitting; runny nose; little appetite for meat; bad digestion; and white and cold skin. Many practitioners have observed that phlegmatic types often possess many of the following qualities: pale, smooth, soft, cold and moist skin; dark blond or blond hair; hairless bodies; shortness of stature; flabby and fat body build; poor appetites; slow or weak digestion; thin and pale urine; pale and loose feces; dreams of water; and apathy.

They often complain of soreness and pain in the lumbar region; loose teeth; deafness and/or tinnitus; thinning and loss of head hair; weakness and pain in the ankles, knees and hips; weakness in hearing and vision; impotence; infertility; miscarriage; and genetic impairments. They may also exhibit growth and development disorders including fertility, conception, and pregnancy problems. Phlegmatic types may suffer from disorders of the central nervous system (MS, muscular dystrophy, or cerebral palsy); diseases of the spinal column, bones, teeth and joints; and disorders in their fluid metabolism.

It is easy to distinguish the various temperaments by watching them eat. At the dinner table, sanguines typically "eat everything in sight;" in a restaurant, they enjoy talking so much that they almost never look at a menu until the waiter arrives. Any sort of stimulants such as sugar, coffee, drugs (even prescription) and, in some cases, wheat and meat products are dangerous for the sanguine type. They (particularly those with excess sanguine) should eat greens daily in the form of Swiss chard, parsley, mint, coriander, chives, argula, rigla, dark greens, and dark green lettuce, and avoid rich or sugary foods.

Sanguine types tend towards yeast infections, fatigue and high nervous system stress because they are typically "abusers" of stimulants, especially sugar and bread. They find that sugar offers a temporary relief during their low cycles, and that bread offers comfort during their high-energy cycles (it slows and cools them down) so they use these substances constantly in a subconscious effort to balance themselves.

When a sanguine person learns to eat more balancing foods in general and to not abuse foods, they will become more balanced themselves and will usually struggle less with yeast infections and other illnesses. When a sanguine person is acting dreamy or "not there," check their sugar consumption or blood sugar levels.

Cholerics seldom vary their menu from one day to another. While eating, they bolt their food down in big chunks, often talking while chewing. Beneficial foods for the choleric type are those that moisturize and cool such as liquids, juicy fruits and vegetables, warm soups, denser root vegetables, sea vegetables, legumes, and fish protein. Raw and cooked foods can be used to balance the choleric's hyper or hypo activity. Warm, cooked foods are stimulating when the choleric is slowed down and tired; cool, raw foods are beneficial when they are overexcited. Cholerics should not eat ice cream, spicy condiments, yogurt, and icy drinks. Adult cholerics should avoid excess curry, sugar, alcohol, caffeine, tea, chili, and salt. Choleric children should avoid colas, sugar, and processed foods.

At the dinner table, melancholics are very picky eaters. It takes them forever to decide what to order at the restaurant but, once it arrives, they savor every bite. The most effective therapies for melancholic excess or ailments involve purging through the use of cleansing fasts or herbs such as senna pods (always use with cinnamon or cumin and limit to, at most, one cup per month). Warming foods, herbs and activities are good for this type.

Phlegmatic types are the most deliberate eaters of all and, invariably, the last ones to finish. This often results in their gaining weight easily because they stay too long at the table, or their being thin because they pick at their food and, because they chew it so well, they may not consume much. They can maintain balance by keeping away from phlegm- inducing foods such as milk, wheat and sweets, eating more heating foods, and engaging in more heating activities. They benefit from the herbs anise, cinnamon, valerian root, fenugreek, cardamom, garlic, and ginger.

The simple observation of excess heat or cold in a person can allow a fairly accurate determination of how to achieve, to a large degree, their healing and health maintenance. In general, you can observe excess heat (the sanguine or choleric element) in a person by noticing the presence of a high fever; feelings of being hot; easy fatigue; excessive thirst; bitter or burning sensations in the mouth; lack of tolerance for hot foods; enjoyment of cold foods and things; and suffering more during the summer or from inflammatory conditions. The person with excess heat or a natural sanguine or choleric temperament should eat cooler foods such as beef; fish; cow's or goat's milk, butter, cheese, and buttermilk; lettuce; celery; sprouts; zucchini; tomato; turnip; cabbage; okra; broccoli; white and sweet potatoes; carrots; cucumbers; apples; melons; pears; figs; apricots; oranges; brown rice; barley; lentils; sunflower oil; green tea; coffee; dill; thyme; rose; vinegar; sour things; and water. They are advised to limit their nuts and seeds, and to engage in "cooling" activities such as praying, meditating, yoga, tai chi, resting, sitting, and reading.

You can observe excess cold (the phlegmatic or melancholic element) in a person if they complain of weak digestion, lack of thirst, catarrhal conditions, suffering most in the winter, and being upset by cold things. They should eat warming foods such as lamb, liver, chicken, goose, duck, eggs, cream cheese, cream, ghee, beets, radishes, onion, mustard greens, leeks, eggplants, red peppers, chick peas, green peppers, turnip, parsley, peaches, plums, limes, lemons, bananas, raisins, dates, figs, olives, dried fruits, sesame seeds, almonds, walnuts, pine nuts, wheat, thin grain rice, basmati rice, sesame oil, black tea, basil, cinnamon, cloves, coriander, garlic, ginger, mint, honey, anise seed, and curry powder. People with excess cold often respond better to sweets and modern medicines than do the other temperaments, who often react badly to them. Phlegmatics or melancholics should also involve themselves in heating activities such as running, walking, intense exercising and other activities, and intense conversations.

Temperamental Depression

by Kristie Karima Burns, Mh, ND

Knowing a person's physiological temperament not only helps to determine the cause of illness, but it also helps in discerning the best treatment. Treating depression is one of the areas in which temperament typing proves invaluable. What constitutes depression varies by temperament type - two people can be exhibiting the same behavior; for one, it may be depression while the other may simply be "in character." Understanding this allows a determination as to the best ways to approach treatment.

There are two popular methods for quickly typing a person's temperament - observing how they eat and how they react to outside stimuli. Pre-determining simply indicates which temperament is strongest in the person.

At the restaurant, sanguines eat everything in sight. They enjoy talking so much that they almost never look at a menu until the waitress arrives. Cholerics are stereotyped eaters; they seldom vary their menu from one day to another. They bolt their food down in big chunks, often talking while chewing. Melancholics are very picky eaters; it takes them forever to make up their minds about what to order, but once it arrives they savor every bite. Phlegmatics are the most deliberate eaters of all and are, invariably, the last ones to finish eating. The sanguine may also be a slow eater, but this is because they are busy playing or being distracted - not because they were concentrating on their food.

In reaction to outside stimuli (a spouse, child, movie, basketball game or party), the sanguine temperament is marked by quick but shallow, superficial excitability; the choleric by quick but strong and lasting; the melancholic temperament by slow but deep; and the phlegmatic by slow but shallow excitability.

Phlegmatics are the ideal type to discuss first as they are often misinterpreted as "lethargically depressed." In reality, however, they are naturally prone to sitting, staring, and living a very moderate and low-key lifestyle. Their needs are fulfilled in this simple and quiet life; in fact, most phlegmatics are completely happy until someone comes along and complains that they are "depressed too much" or that they "lack ambition" or that "something is wrong because they sit around too much." Then, they may end up sitting around considering that they just might be depressed. They will soon have themselves convinced that they are, and may even come up with some very valid reasons as to why. Oftentimes, they will be labeled (by themselves as well as by others) as depressed for no other reason except that they fall into this type. However, the reality of the situation with the phlegmatic is that they are naturally unenthusiastic and immobile by nature.

If this quality is understood and accepted by them and those around them, all can live happily with their slow and steady attitude about life. Eeyore, from the cartoon "Winnie the Pooh," is a good example of this type of person. Thankfully, his friends in the Hundred Acre Woods are wise enough not to get him treated for depression.

Sanguine types, on the other hand, are the last people you would expect to get depressed. They are the people who display the most joy and enthusiasm for life. Sanguines are also the people who often start new projects while stumbling over old ones so that they can manage to fit in all the wonderful things they want to do. However, life is not all smiles for sanguines as they are prone to seasonal depressions (SAD in particular) and mood swings (during PMS, hypoglycemic attacks, etc.). Their life perceptions and moods come in cycles like the seasons; their internal seasons rotating as they are influenced by the external seasons so they may find themselves suddenly depressed because of the weather, a lack of sun or fresh air, or simply the change of seasons.

Sanguine types are also very influenced by foods, which often effect their internal cycles. Many times, they become depressed after eating foods that they are allergic to or after consuming too much caffeine, processed foods, or sugar. Sanguines tend to blame themselves for their depression; acutely aware that they are no longer being their "lovable and cheerful" self, they often "hide" until they are "done" being depressed. Because people usually enjoy them for their vibrancy, they are not usually enthusiastic about sharing any feelings of depression and they may have a hard time asking for help. You may not hear from a sanguine friend for a few days or even weeks at a time, and then she may suddenly appear again as if no time has passed. However, in most cases a sanguine's depression is seasonal or passing, or can be cured by regulating their diet. In many cases, recognizing their condition as natural and normal for their type and just "waiting for the storm to pass" is the best "cure." Tigger, in "Winnie the Pooh," is a perfect example of the sanguine type. Melancholic types tend to get depressed more easily than any of the others. Although the phlegmatic may constantly LOOK depressed, the melancholic suffers from an almost constant self-induced depression caused by their over-evaluation and reflection on life. They usually do not let one thing go unnoticed and everything cumulates to depress their spirits about life. ine However, treating a melancholic for depression is often destructive, as they are melancholy by nature and even gain some joy and satisfaction from dwelling on their life miseries. You will usually find that melancholics are even more depressed when nothing is wrong in their life as they enjoy solving problems and overcoming challenges. The most depressed melancholic is one who is having a day where nothing went wrong at work, home or anywhere else in their life - leaving them with a feeling of dread about what could possibly come next. The best way for a melancholic to deal with depression is for them to learn to laugh at themselves. They will always be a little "depressed" so they should avoid using the label "depressed," instead, they should describe their feelings differently so they don't take themselves so seriously. They can state instead that they feel "a little melancholy" today," which is more appropriate and completely normal - there is no reason to "cure" a person of a little melancholy. In fact, the worst thing a melancholic can do is indulge in their depression by giving it a name and then "treating it." Usually, the process of naming their feelings depression and then feeding it through treatment just creates a sense of satisfaction and justification for their feelings. A typical melancholic would be happy to be on medication their entire life. Winnie the Pooh is a good example of a melancholic person. He is easily influenced by the suggestion that something might be wrong, and he is constantly saying, "oh, bother."

Choleric types rarely get depressed; when they do, it is usually because of a loss or some other external factor, and it is typically dramatic - they may wail, "I am so depressed" for a period of time and then go on to something more interesting. Depression for the choleric consists of immobility, lethargy or moping, but includes movement and drama. The problem with this is that they may actually enjoy and benefit from the drama to some extent, but those around them may easily become infected by their mood of despair.

The typical choleric can act dramatically and hysterically depressed, create a feeling of depression in those around them, and then move on to other things while the people they have "infected" remain depressed. The best way to deal with a depressed choleric is to quarantine them from other people, and engage them in physical work or exercise. Hiking in the hills, running, swimming, and Tai Chi are all good for this type. Instead of using up all that dramatic energy in a state of depression, they need to use it in sports and it will gradually dissipate without harming anyone around them. Rabbit, from "Winnie the Pooh," is a good example of this type of person. When he is depressed or upset, he wails out loud — infecting the entire clan with his mood and oftentimes scaring Pooh and his friends away from his house or garden.

Above all, remember that giving a name to depression is often the cause of the problem. Some temperament types are naturally more low-key; some people function in cycles and will experience some form of depression at least once a year while others are naturally more melancholic than others, and yet others tend to be dramatic about their depression and enjoy the attention their drama brings.

In short, depression is probably more natural than unnatural; rather than being a stigmatic problem, it should be viewed as more of a normal occurrence. Depression CAN be crippling, causing people to lie in bed, skip work or school, end relationships and even contemplate suicide. It should be taken seriously; however, helping people to get in touch with their inner natures can help THEM to take it less seriously and, perhaps, lead them to being healed.

Humeral Properties of Foods and Herbs

by Kristie Karima Burns, Mh, ND

Food or Herb	Hot & Dry Choleric	Hot & Wet Sanguine	Neutral	Cold & Dry Melancholic	Cold & Wet Phlegmatic
Acacia	Acacia				
Aloe Vera					Aloe Vera
Anise	Anise				
Apple				Apple	
Apricot			Apricot		
Apricot Seed		Apricot Seed			
Asparagus				Asparagus	
Balm of Gilead		Balm of Gilead			
Banana				Banana	
Basil	Basil				
Barberry				Barberry	
Barley				Barley	
Beef		Beef			
Beet		Beet			
Black Pepper	Black Pepper				
Black Sesame			Black Sesame		
Borage					Borage
Brown Sugar		Brown Sugar			
Butter		Butter			
Camphor					Camphor
Caroway	Caroway				
Cardamom		Cardamom			
Carrot		Carrot			
Catnip	Catnip				
Celandine	Celandine				
Celery		Celery			
Chamomile	Chamomile				
Cherry		Cherry			
Chestnut					Chestnut
Chickory	Chickory				
Chicken		Chicken			
Chicken Egg		Chicken Egg			
Egg White				Egg White	
Egg Yolk		Egg Yolk			
Chicory			Chicory		
Chives	Chives				
Cinnamon	Cinnamon				
Clam					Clam
Clove	Clove				
Coconut		Coconut			
Coffee		Coffee			
Comfrey				Comfrey	
Coriander	Coriander				
Corn		Corn			
Crab					Crab

76

Food or Herb	Hot & Dry	Hot & Wet	Neutral	Cold & Dry	Cold & Wet
Cucumber			Cucumber		
Cumin	Cumin				
Date		Date			
Dill	Dill				
Duck				Duck	
Eggplant			Eggplant		
Fennel	Fennel				
Fenugreek	Fenugreek				
Fig		Fig			
Frankincense	Frankinsense				
Garlic	Garlic				
Gentian				Gentian	
Ginger	Ginger				
Ginseng		Ginseng			
Goldenseal	Goldenseal				
Grapefruit				Grapefruit	
Grapes			Grapes		
Guava		Guava			
Green Pepper	Green Pepper				
Henna					Henna
Honey		Honey			
Hops					Hops
Horehound	Horehound				
Hyssop					Hyssop
Jasmine				Jasmine	
Juniper				Juniper	
Kelp					Kelp
Kidneys (beef)		Beef Kidney			
Kidneys-sheep		Kidney-Sheep			
Lavender	Lavender				
Leek	Leeks				
Lemon		Lemon			
Lettuce				Lettuce	
Licorice		Licorice			
Linseed (Flax)					Flax (Linseed)
Liver (Beef)		Liver (beef)			
Liver (chicken)		Liver (Chick)			
Liver (sheep)				Liver (sheep)	
Lobelia	Lobelia				
Malt		Malt			
Mandarins				Mandarins	
Mango				Mango	
Marjorum		Marjorum			
Marshmallow		Marshmallow			
Milk (cow)		Milk (cow)			
Milk (sheep)		Milk (sheep)			
Mugwort	Mugwort				
Mung Bean			Mung Bean		
Muskmelon				Musklmelon	

Food or Herb	Hot & Dry	Hot & Wet	Neutral	Cold & Dry	Cold & Wet
Mustard	Mustard				
Mutton		Mutton			
Myrrh				Myrrh	
Myrtle				Myrtle	
Nigella Sativa	Nigella Sativa				
Nutmeg	Nutmeg				
Olive			Olive		
Oysters				Oysters	
Papaya		Papaya			
Peach		Peach			
Peanut		Peanut			
Pear				Pear	
Peppermint		Peppermint			
Persimmon				Persimmon	
Pinneapple			Pinneapple		
Pistachio	Pistachio				
Plantain				Plantain	
Plum			Plum		
Pomegranate				Pomegranate	
Poppy Seed				Poppy Seed	
Potato				Potato	
Pumpkin			Pumpkin		
Purslane					Purslane
Rasidh		Radish			
Rasberry		Rasberry			
Red Clover	Red Clover				
Red Pepper	Red Pepper				
Rhubarb	Rhubarb				
Rose				Rose	
Rosemary	Rosemary				
Saffron		Saffron			
Salt					Salt
Sandalwood				Sandalwood	
Sarsparilla	Sarsparilla				
Seaweed					Seaweed
Senna	Senna				
Sesame Oil			Sesame Oil		
Shallots	Shallots				
Shrimp		Shrimp			
Soybean		Soybean			
Squaw Vine	Squaw Vine				
Spearmint	Spearmint				
Spinach			Spinach		
Squash		Squash			
Star Anise	Star Anise				
Star Fruit				Star Fruit	
Strawberry				Strawberry	
String Beans		String Beans			
Sumac				Sumac	

Food or Herb	Hot & Dry	Hot & Wet	Neutral	Cold & Dry	Cold & Wet
Sugar Cane				Sugar Cane	
Sunflowerseed		Sunflowerseed			
Sweet Potato				Sweet Potato	
Tangerine				Tangerine	
Tobacco	Tobacco				
Tofu			Tofu		
Tomato				Tomato	
Turmeric	Turmeric				
Valerian	Valerian				
Vinegar				Vinegar	
Walnuts				Walnuts	
Watermelon					Watermelon
Wheat			Wheat		
Wheat Bran			Wheat Bran		
White Sugar		White Sugar			
Wild Rue				Wild Rue	
Yams		Yams			

Word Comparison Chart of The Four Humors in Healing, Nutrition and Personality

by Kristie Karima Burns, MH, ND

Diagnosis of Underlying Type

	Hot & Wet	Hot & Dry	Cold & Dry	Cold & Wet
Humor	Blood	Yellow Bile	Black Bile	Phlegm
Personality	Sanguine	Choleric	Melancholic	Phlemnatic
Chinase	Wood	Fire	Metal	Water
Greek Element	Air/Wind	Fire	Earth	Water
Avurvedic Element	Vatta	Pitta	NONE	Kapha

The Four Humors

Age	Childhood	Youth	Maturity	Old Age
Animals	Monkey	Bear	Owl	Dolphin
Appetite	N/A	Poor	Faulty Cravings	N/A
Archetype	Purpose	Fulfillment	Order	Truth
Av. Excretion	Saliva	Sweat Tears	Feces	Urine
Avicenna Organ	Circulation	Liver	Skeleton	Muscles
Celestine	Poor me	Intimidator	Interrogator	Aloof
Ch. Excretion	Tears	Sweat	Mucus	Sexual

Charlie Brown	Snoopy	Lucy	Linus	Charlie Brown
Chinese Organ	Liver	Heart Network	Lung Network	Kidney
Color	Aquamarine	Red	White	Purple
Comics	Snoopy	Jason	Ziggy	Cathy
Desires	Purpose	Fulfillment	Order	Truth
Dimensions	Movement	Space	Shape	Time
Dreads	Confinement	Gravity	Crowding	Invasion
Dreams	Sees Red Things Blood etc	Sees Fires-Yellow Flags Yellow Objects, the Sun	Fear of Darkness terrifying black things	Sees Waters river snow
E.E. Milne	Tigger	Rabbit	Eeyore/Gopher	Pooh/Piglet
Enneagram	Helper Romantic	Adventurer Achiever	Asserter Perfectionist	Peacemaker Observer
Expression	Anger	Joy	Sorrow	Fear
Feel of Skin	Film	NA	Rough & Hard	Solf & Cool
Flavor	Sour	Bitter	Spicy	Salty
Fromm (1947)	Exploiting	Hoarding	Marketing	Receptive
Geometrics (78)	Squiggle	Triangle	Square	Circle
Hair	Normal	Hairy	Hairy Absent	Chest
Injury from	Wind	Heat	Dry	Cold
Jung	Feeler	Sensor	Thinker	Intuitor
Keirsy (1967)	Artisan, Sensation Seeking	Guardian Security Seeking	Rational Knowledge Seeking	Idealist Identity Seeking
Kretschner (1920)	Hyomanic	Melancholic	Hyperashetic	Anesthetic
Meyers-Briggs	SP	NT	SJ	NF
Mouth	Canker Sores	Bitter Taste	N/A	Sticky Saliva
Odor	Rancid	Acrid	Fishy	Rotten

Path	Action	Compassion	Mastery	Knowledge
Physique	Good Lean	Joints Large	Emaciated	Effeminate
Plato (340 BC)	Artisan	Guardian	Scientist	Philosopher
Power	Expansion	Fusion	Contraction	Consolidation
PSI	Promoter	Controller	Analyst	Supporter
Region	East	South	West	North
Season	Spring	Summer	Autumn	Winter
Sense	Hearing	Smell	Touch	Taste
Skin	Flushed	Yellowish Tinge	Dark & Hairy	Pale & Weak
Sprangler (1930)	Aesthetic	Religious	Economic	Theoretic
Tends to	Risk stay busy	Seek excitement	Make judgments	Seek solitude
Time	Dawn	Noon	Dusk	Midnight
Tongue	Red	Rough & Dry	N/A	N/A
True Colors (78)	Orange	Green	Gold	Blue
Types A & B	Type B Messy	Type B Motivated	Type A Compulsive	Type A Casual
Urine	N/A	N/A	Dark Colored	White
Virtue	Fervor	Charisma	Righteousness	Honesty
Voice	Hollering	Giggling	Sobbing	Groaning

Detecting Imbalance Seen from Chinese Point of View

Exaggerated

Domination	Inmolation	Restriction	Negation
High Blood Pressure	Enlarged Heart	Overexpanded Chest	Hypersensative
Oily Skin & Hair	Sweating	Dry cough	Tight Chest
Headaches	Boils	Flushed Fase	Sinus Headache above
Cramps – long muscles	Chest pain	Nasal Polyps	Lack of Sweat
Vertigo	Painful Urination	Dry Hair & Skin Scalp	Lack of Urine
Ringing in the Ears	Erratics Pulse Strong	No Sweat	Hardening of blood
Constipation w/cramps	Overheated	Stiff spine & neck	Sciatica
Sores of mouth &	Large pores & cartlage	Pain in the Ribs	Pulmonary hypert
Constipation	Rigid Joints	Heartburn	Dry painful eczema
Dry cracked nails	Bony tumors	Difficult Swallow	Easy sexual excitement
Scanty urine	Weak digestion	Eye/ear pain	But difficult to please
Dry nose-throat	Precocious Sex	Shingles	Weak Digestion
Accident prone	Shrink gums	Hard, thick Nails	Little Sleep
Breast pain	Tendon Injury	Constipation	Hypertension

Collapsed

Compression	Disintegration	Constriction	Petrification
Labile Blood Pressure	Slow Pulse	Narrow Chest	Dulled Vision
Hypoglycemia	Irregular Pulse	Frail Physique	Dulled Hearing
Blurry Vision	Weak Heart	Short of Breath	Ringing in Ears
Sensitive to Light	Chills Easily	Incontinence	Weak & Stiff Spine and Joints
Sesitive to Sound	Overheats easily	Congestion	Cystitis
Low Blood Pressure	Moles & Warts	Itchy Eyes	Anemic
Headaches from disc problems	Tendonitis	Fainst or Dizzy easily	Sadness
Cold buttocks	Dry Nails	Tired easily	Loss of body hair
Frequent Uriniation	Lax joints	Excitement	Cracked Nails
Osteoporosis	Tense Muscles	Premature Orgasm	Soft Nails
Premature Gray	Irritable Colon	Enlarged Lymph Nodes	Infertility
Lacks Stamina	Hard to Wake	Loss of Appetite	

Common

PMS	Sleep Disorders	Respiratory Disorders	Memory Problems
Lateral Headaches	Heart/Arteries	Skin Ailments	Alertness
Migraine	Heart Rate Disturbances	Dehydration	Distorted
TMJ	Disturbances of Speech	Elimination	Bones & Teeth
Facial Neuralgia	Blood Pressure & Circulation Issues	Venous Circulation	Cysts
Hypertension	Circulation Issues	Lymphatic Circulation Problems	Disrupted Sleep Patterns
Sexual Dysfunction	Lymphatic Circulation Patterns	Painful Menses	Substance Abuse

Detecting Imbalance from Avicenna's Point of View

Headache	Headache	Headache	Headache
Delirium	Delirium	Delirium	Lethargy
Lethargy	Insomnia	Stiffness	Lethargy
Weak Limbs	Nose Itching	Insomnia	Melancholy
Nose Itching	Hard Eyelids	Hallucinations	Madness
Poor Vision	Boils on Eyelids	Cankar Sores	Forgetfulness
Enlarged Tongue	Canker Sores	Diphtheria	Paralysis
Canker Sores	Dull Teeth	Cancer	Weak Limbs
Swollen Palate	Discolored Teeth	Excessive Appetite	Convulsions
Trembling Lips	Coughing	Swollen Stomach	Muscular Tense
Loose Teeth	Pleurisy	Vomiting	Trembling Lips
Tooth Spaces	Feeling of Smoke in Chest	Heartburn	Trembling
Diptheria	Heart Attack	Swelling of Liver	Swollen Lids
Slackness Uvula	Excessive Appetite	Jaundice	Shedding Lash
Pleurisy	Swelling of Liver	Flatulence	Styes
Swelling of Liver	Jaundice	Arthritis	Pupils Dilated
Hemorrhoids	Hemorrhoids	Gripe Eyelid	Dandruff
Swollen Testicles	Gripe	Bladder Swelling	Odor From Nose
Constant Errection	Anal Ulcer	Ringing in Ears	Colic
Convulsion of Penis	Burning Urination	Excessive Libido	Enlarge Tongue

Cracked Nails	Swollen Testicles	Swelling of Womb	Bad Breath
Excessive Menses	Varicose Veins	Canker Sores	Yellow Nails
Thickened Nails	Swollen Palate	Skin Cancer	White Lips
Swelling of Lips	Dull Feel Teeth	Gum Ulcers	Swelling Uvula
Diptheria	Constriction in Throat	Asthma	Coughing
Pleurisy	Heart feel pulled downward	Deficient Appetite	Severe Thrist
Vomiting	Upset Stomach	Convulsion of Stomach	Liver Obstruct
Liver Swell	Itching Anus	Gripe	Colic
Kidney Ulcer	Constipation	Bladder Swell	Urine Retain
Inability to get errection	Excessive Menses	Swelling of Womb	Backache
Joint ache	Arthritis	Sebaceaus	Cyst
Pimples	Acne	Balness	No nail growth
Boils	Scabs	Dandruff	Sweat

Assignment for Section Three

1. Choose four people. Decide which temperament they are.
2. Using the Chinese and Avicenna part of the chart figure out what temperament their ailment is. Example: If they have a fever, sore throat and cough look under the various types to see where these three symptoms are listed. In this case the disease would be type: Choleric. List the type under the personality type
3. Look at your list. The two types may be the same or different. Figure out what is in imbalance here. Do you have a hot person who has a hot disease? Then you need to cool them down. Look at the elements that are in play here and use foods and herbs to balance your "client". Keep in mind that if you have a person with a cold temperament and they have a hot ailment that they still need cooling down. If the person you are evaluating has no ailment you can still use herbs and foods to balance their temperament. Thus, a child or person with a HOT temperament can be made calmer with cooler foods and herbs. A person with a COLD temperament can be made more active and alert with hot foods, etc...
4. To find out the herbs and foods to use for balancing you need to consult this chapter and the chart that categorizes herbs and foods according to their properties of Hot, Cold, Moist or Dry.

~Section Four: Diets for Healing~

Detox/ Healing Signs

When doing any detox program you will find that on the fourth, seventh or tenth day you will experience a "healing crisis". This occurs because your body is throwing off the toxins you have accumulated in your body into your system so they can be eliminated. This means that until you do eliminate them they will be once again in your blood and digestive tract causing you a worsening of symptoms and/or symptoms of cold, flu or other misery. This is why exercise and bowel movements are so important during fasting. Your goal is to get the body to release the toxins it is storing and then to EXPEL these toxins. This expelling will be accomplished through sweating and bowel movements usually although in some people they will get vomiting or asthma and expel toxins through other methods (this is rare though). You need to exercise not just for the sweating, but also to help move the toxins DOWN so they can be eliminated. Walking for 20 minutes a day is fine. You also need to be sure to drink 8-10 glasses of fluid a day so they toxins are diluted and able to move out of your system. You WILL experience a healing crisis as you heal, if you are really healing. So do not be alarmed at any worsening or symptoms that initially appear.

TIP: Please remember to eat A LOT. When you are detoxing on vegetables, juices and teas you need to eat every 2-3 hours and you also need to eat MORE than you normally would. You will not gain weight by eating more and more often. You will probably still lose weight, but if you do not eat often enough or prepare enough food you will be weak and hungry and the detox will be difficult and less effective.

Healing Crisis as a Welcome Sign

The phenomenon of the **"healing crisis"** is not discussed much in health circles these days. However, the concept is as relevant today as it was 100 years ago when it first began to appear in Western literature. An understanding of healing crises could, in fact, be beneficial to many who are now embarking on the path of healing. This reaction can be strong or mild, but it must and will manifest. Knowing that a healing crisis is inevitable, and having some idea of the ways in which it might manifest, will, at the very least, prepare a patient for its arrival and may also offer some comfort through the duration of the "crisis."

Generally, a healing crisis initiates when a person who is undergoing some form of natural therapy experiences some improvement. The patient feels better and stronger, both physically and mentally. Then, without warning, the old illness or even symptoms of by-gone illnesses reappear. When this happens, most patients become confused and discouraged, believing that all the progress they had made is now lost and that they must start over or give up. However, that is far from what is really occurring. Anyone who has ever experienced any form of chronic illness or condition, whether internal, such as an ulcer, or structural, such as a long-term back disability, can attest to the fact that there is a loss of energy associated with the illness.

Lack of vitality always accompanies chronic health conditions, and this energy loss limits or even prevents healing. The body is stuck in a rut, so to speak; it is unable to garner its forces sufficiently to restore well-being.

When improvement occurs, vitality is restored to the body, and its self-healing mechanisms are awakened. As healing begins, symptoms reappear as part of the body's process of eliminating diseased cells and toxins from its tissues. Hence the assessment that the healing crisis is actually good news because it is a sign and signal of deep healing and restoration. It should be added that, not surprisingly, the patient always feels better after the healing crisis has run its course.

The healing crisis is recognized today by many natural health practitioners. Homeopaths call these incidents "aggravations" and chiropracters refer to the phenomenon as "retracing." What is important for us to understand is that a healing crisis, or any healing that will sustain us over the long haul, must occur at some point in the therapeutic program. It can help to know what, in general, to anticipate. In addition to the reactivation of old symptoms, a patient might also feel unexpectedly exhausted, experience flu-like symptoms, or feel achiness all over the body. These symptoms usually pass in 24 to 48 hours and the patient will feel stronger in some way after the event. Natural Healers have also noted that the body has a definite priority and pattern of using its own healing energy to get well. A famous American homeopath, Constantine Herring, MD., formulated a theory (known as the Herring Law of Cure) which says that the healing energy awakens first at the deepest level, then moves to the surface where it begins healing the body from head to toe. In a similar priority, the body's healing mechanism will attend to the most current illness first and move through to the oldest (historically) last. In other words (as stated in the Law of Cure), disease is healed "from the inside out, from the head down, and in the reverse order that it appeared." Daniel David Palmer, DC., founder of chiropractic, often quoted this theory which he described as the "ADIOS Principle" in health restoration, "adios" being an acronym for "above, down, inside, out."

It should also be mentioned that old mental or emotional symptoms may re-activate during a healing crisis. Dr. R.H. Van Wyck, Director of the Vancouver Institute for Applied Psychology has stated, "Each physical state is accompanied by a psychological counterpart and strictly psychotrauma or heavy emotional material is also re-experienced during the reversal and healing process."

Healing crises are very welcome signs when we experience them. Unfortunately, in today's world, these "aggravations" or "retracings" do not occur as frequently as they did in the past. The intense social and economic stresses facing most people today, as well as the toxic load in the environment, often stand in the body's way and prevent a restoration of vitality needed to initiate a healing crisis.

The obstacles are many, but the potential is still there for a healing crisis. Understanding that these "aggravations" or "retracings" are part of the recovery process de-mystifies natural health. When such an event appears, we can then welcome it rather than suppress it.

Blood Building Diet

- 75% of this diet is fruits and vegetables - *30% of this is raw*
- Grains, nuts, seeds, meat, fish and poultry are the other 25%
- Processed and synthetic foods are non-existent: this includes anything in a box or can, candy, coffee, chocolate, sugar, etc...
- The only oil to be used is olive oil in small quantities.
- Use minimal salt.
- Meals
  - Breakfast: Fruit only
  - Lunch: Starch meal
  - Evening: Protein meal
  - Snacks: raw vegetables only or freshly made juices, green food supplements

Daily Schedule
- Pre-Breakfast: Water: Tea
- Breakfast
  - Saturday: orange and grapefruit with dates
  - Sunday: orange and pineapple with dates
  - Monday: apples and banana with figs
  - Tuesday: dark grapes and apricots
  - Wednesday: figs, dates, dark grapes and red apples
  - Thursday: Black currants or raisins with apples
  - Friday: pomegranate and banana with raisins or figs or dates
- Snack: Green supplement: Green herbal tea (2 tsp. Herb)
- Starch Meals, any vegetable combination with any grain like:
  - Saturday: Salad with shredded beets, carrots & peas in tomato sauce over a baked potato as the starch
  - Sunday: Salad with spinach or gargir, cauliflower and broccoli stir fry over brown rice as the starch
  - Monday: Vegetable salad with chard (red and green), green squash with fresh corn as the starch
  - Tuesday: Vegetable salad with beets, vegetable stew with whole grain bread as the starch
  - Wednesday: Vegetable salad with spinach or dark green, vegetable stew, sweet potato as a starch
  - Thursday: Vegetable salad with chard, vegetable soup with barley
  - Friday: Vegetable salad with gargir, tabbouli, vegetable casserole with brown rice or brown bread
- Snack: Green supplement: Green herbal tea (2 tsp. Herb)
- Protein Meals, any vegetable combination with any meat or protein like eggs, cheese or nuts, chicken, liver or beef. However, you are only allowed ONE PROTEIN A MEAL, you cannot combine yogurt with meat or any two proteins or anything like that. Here is a weekly schedule:
  - Saturday: Vegetable salad, okra vegetable main dish, spinach, pine nuts, beef liver
  - Sunday: Vegetable salad, beets, chicken soup with herbs and parsley, chicken.

- o Monday: Vegetable salad, green beans with beef stew, gargir
- o Tuesday: Vegetable salad, Chard, stir fry with broccoli, boiled eggs or omelet
- o Wednesday: Vegetable salad, cauliflower & green beans stir fry, chicken liver with onions
- o Thursday: Vegetable salad with fresh spinach or gargir, fish and vegetable dish
- o Friday: Vegetable salad with fresh spinach or gargir, beets, and your choice of meat or cheese, nuts or yogurt
- Snack
  - o Green supplement
  - o Green herbal tea (2 tsp. Herb)

General Rules
- Begin each meal with a raw food (vegetable salad)
- Eat fruit separate from other things and do not combine with other foods or meals
- Do not drink water or other drinks with the meal
- Do not drink milk or eat cheese. Use only yogurt in small quantities with the evening meal some days but not all days.
- Do not eat proteins and starches together (bread and meat or bread with cheese or a baked potato with meat) EVER!

Give yourself three days to one week to adapt and then continue for three weeks on this "diet". The only thing this diet eliminates is processed foods, unnatural fats and oils, sugar and pure milk. It allows you all other foods within limits so you are not being deprived, you are simply limiting and re-proportioning for a while.

Foods to Avoid
- Coffee
- Sugar
- White Flour
- Packaged or canned foods (frozen is OK)
- Tea with Caffeine
- Sodas
- Synthetic or restaurant foods
- Green Tea (with caffeine)
- Nettles
- Alfalfa
- Horsetail
- Boneset
- Red Clover

Optional Foods
- Lycium Berries
- Alma
- Bilberry
- Black Currants
- Mulberry Fruit

Balancing Diet (Anti-Acid Diet)

- 75% Fruits and vegetables - *30% is raw*
- 25% Grains, nuts, seeds, meat, fish and poultry
- Processed and synthetic foods are non-existent: this includes anything in a box or can, candy, coffee, chocolate, sugar, etc...
- The only oil to be used is olive oil in small quantities.
- Use minimal salt.
- Meals
    - Breakfast: Fruit only
    - Lunch: Starch meal
    - Evening: Protein meal
    - Snacks: vegetables only or freshly made juices

Daily Schedule
- Breakfast
    - Orange and grapefruit
    - Orange and pineapple
    - Grapefruit and sour apples
    - Bananas, pears, dates, sweet grapes
    - Figs, dates, sweet grapes, sweet apples
- Starch Meals, any vegetable combination with any grain like:
    - Vegetable salad, carrots, potatoes, beets
    - Vegetable salad, asparagus, brown rice, cauliflower
    - Vegetable salad, green squash, fresh corn, asparagus
    - Vegetable salad, squash, okra, whole grain bread
    - Vegetable salad, broccoli, chard, kale, sweet potatoes etc.
- Protein Meals, any vegetable combination with any meat or protein like beans, tofu, eggs, cheese or nuts. However, you are only allowed ONE PROTEIN A MEAL, you cannot combine yogurt with meat or buts with tofu or anything like that. Also you must make a weekly rotation and make sure you rotate:
    - Monday: Beans or tofu
    - Tuesday: Beef
    - Wednesday: yogurt
    - Thursday: Eggs
    - Friday: Chicken
    - Saturday: Fish, tuna, or salmon or other fish
    - Sunday: Any of the above repeated or something different like turkey or quail or lamb
    - Vegetable salad, green squash, spinach, nuts
    - Vegetable salad, yellow squash, cabbage, sunflower seeds
    - Vegetable salad, green beans, kale, cottage cheese or labna
    - Vegetable salad, Swiss Chard, broccoli, eggs
    - Vegetable salad, cauliflower, green beans, roast chicken/beef or turkey or fish

General Rules
- Begin each meal with a raw food (vegetable salad)
- Eat fruit separate from other things and do not combine with other foods or meals
- Do not drink water or other drinks with the meal
- Do not drink milk or eat cheese. Use only yogurt in small quantities with the evening meal some days but not all days.
- Do not eat proteins and starches together (bread and meat or bread with cheese or baked potato with meat) EVER!

Give yourself three days to one week to adapt and then continue for three weeks on this "diet". The only thing this diet eliminates is processed foods, unnatural fats and oils, sugar and pure milk. It allows you all other foods within limits so you are not being deprived, you are simply limiting and re-proportioning for a while.

Foods to Avoid
- Coffee
- Sugar
- White Flour
- Packaged or canned foods (frozen is OK)
- Tea with Caffeine
- Sodas
- Synthetic or restaurant foods

Candida Diet

- 75% of diet Fruits and vegetables are - *30% of this is raw*
- 25%Grains, nuts, seeds, meat, fish and poultry are the other
- Processed and synthetic foods are non-existent: this includes anything in a box or can, candy, coffee, chocolate, sugar, etc...
- The only oil to be used is olive oil in small quantities.
- Use minimal salt.
- Meals
  - Breakfast: Fruit only
    ** Avoid the very juicy and the dried fruits
  - Lunch: Starch meal
    ** Avoid wheat and oats more than once a week
    ** Avoid potatoes and corn or minimize to once a week. Emphasize greens. Minimize mushrooms.
  - Evening: Protein meal
    ** Avoid potatoes and corn or minimize to once a week. Emphasize greens. Minimize mushrooms.
    ** Do not eat beef or milk products
  - Snacks: vegetables only
    ** Avoid potatoes and corn or minimize to once a week. Emphasize greens

Daily Schedule

- Breakfast, avoid all very juicy fruits and dried fruits which can be moldy. Avoid melons and oranges. Peel all fruit. Eat it fresh only and no frozen.
  - Apples - two kinds
  - Mango & kiwi
  - Papaya & Pineapple Apples - two kinds
  - Pears & Peaches
  - Kiwi & Mango
  - Papaya and Pineapple
- Starch Meals, any vegetable combination with any grain like:
  - Brown Basmati Rice and vegetable
  - Barley and vegetable
  - Potatoes and vegetable sauce
  - Butternut Squash and vegetable
  - Brown Basmati Rice and vegetable
  - Barley and vegetable
  - Oats and vegetable
  -

Do not use ANY wheat products and go easy with the oats.

- Protein Meals, any vegetable combination with any meat or protein like beans, tofu, eggs, cheese or nuts. However, you are only allowed **ONE PROTEIN A MEAL**, you cannot combine yogurt with meat or buts with tofu or anything like that. Also you must make a weekly rotation and make sure you rotate:
    - Monday: Eggs with turnips
    - Tuesday: Fish with tomatoes
    - Wednesday: turkey or chicken with broccoli
    - Thursday: lamb or veal with cabbage
    - Friday: Eggs with avacado
    - Saturday: Fish with greens
    - Sunday: Turkey or chicken with greens

General Rules

- Begin each meal with a raw food (vegetable salad)
- Eat fruit separate from other things and do not combine with other foods or meals
- Do not drink water or other drinks with the meal
- Do not drink milk or eat cheese. Use only yogurt in small quantities with the evening meal some days but not all days.
- Do not eat proteins and starches together (bread and meat or bread with cheese or a baked potato with meat) EVER!

Give yourself three days to one week to adapt and then continue for three weeks on this "diet". The only thing this diet eliminates is processed foods, unnatural fats and oils, sugar and pure milk. It allows you all other foods within limits so you are not being deprived, you are simply limiting and re-proportioning for a while.

Foods to Avoid
- Coffee
- Sugar
- White Flour
- Packaged or canned foods (frozen is OK)
- Tea with Caffeine
- Sodas
- Synthetic or restaurant food

10-Day Detox Fast

Allowed

- Vegetables: Asparagus, beet, broccoli, Brussel sprouts, carrot, celery, Swiss chard, cucumber, eggplant, endive, garlic, kholrabi, lettuce, mushroom, mustard greens, onion, parsley, parsnip, pepper, potato, radish, spinach, squash, tomato, watercress (argula.)
- Legumes: Beans (green or snap), peas.
- Grains and flours: Wheat germ, bran, oatmeal.
- Fruits: Avocado
- Seeds: Pumpkin, squash, sesame, sunflower.
- Nuts: Brazil (for protein), pinon.
- Meats: If you MUST, have only 3-5 ounces of chicken breast per day or fish.
- Dairy products: Yogurt (maximum one cup a day.)
- Herbs: Chives, sweet basil, dill.
- Drinks: Green herb teas like chamomile, peppermint, alfalfa, nettles, etc.

Foods to Avoid
- Oil
- Salt
- MSG
- Milk
- Tea
- Candy
- Snacks
- Bread
- Sugar
- Honey

Do not use Maggi or other Chicken bouillon cubes to cook with during this time. Use only fresh vegetable broth, water or homemade chicken broth.

Ideas
- Stir Fry vegetables
- Chop veggies in a pot and bake them in a tomato or other sauce for 30 minute in a covered pan
- Use oatmeal to thicken soups and sauces, then blend some in the blender for a creamy soup.
- Slice vegetables in fingers and steam or bake with curry powder or fresh herbs
- Zucchini and carrots with fresh dill
- Potatoes with chives, garlic and onions
- Potatoes with fresh dill and a bit of mustard
- Bisilla, bemia, fusulia all made without oil and no rice
- Soups
- Oatmeal - plain (for kids with apple and raisin)
- Raw vegetables cut up
- Chopped salads with lettuce, tomato, onion, broccoli, cauliflower, peppers, and carrots.

- Zucchini and tomato stir fry with chopped spinach or parsley and Italian season
- Tomato Soup with green pepper, carrot and squash
- Broccoli and cauliflower stir fry

Cooking Tips
- For oil in cooking use broth or water or a little butter or a tsp. of olive oil only.
- Do not use salt. Don't worry. After two days your food will taste naturally salty.
- Use yogurt in soups and cooking for a creamy effect and in place of oil for baba ganoush.
- Use only plain yogurt.
- Each person gets only 1 small chicken BREAST a day or fish or no meat. No more!
- Chop up carrots, celery, broccoli, cauliflower, etc. and keep them in a container for when anyone gets hungry.
- Keep a basket of apples and oranges out for the children when they get hungry.
- Use any leftover stir fries for soups the next day.
- Use a lot of fresh herbs or spices to make up for the lack of salt.
- Make a glass of carrot or carrot celery juice for a snack. (You can add an apple to the juice to make it sweeter but it must all be homemade juice.)
- Make it simple! Make oatmeal for breakfast with mint tea and then soup and chicken and salad for lunch. When you are stuck make soup or raw veggies.
- Buy some canned peas and carrots, beets and green beans for quick snacks-emergency hunger.
- Preplan your meals and think about what you will make all week before you start. This will make shopping and cooking easier to plan. Don't worry about making the same thing more than once.
- Drink a lot of water.
- Plan to eat a small nibble of veggies, glass of carrot juice or apple between the meals so you will not be hungry. Plan ahead! Perhaps prepare some meals, shop and plan for two days before you start.

Must
- Walk every day to sweat.
- Shower or bathe daily with loufa.
- Drink lots of water, 8-10 glasses.

21-Day Green Drink Fast

Daily Schedule

- Pre-Breakfast, one glass of water after waking up
- Breakfast , 30 minutes after pre-breakfast have 1 to 2 pieces of fruit
- Snack, have 1-2 cups of zucchini, dandelion <leaves>, potato and apple juice with 1 TBS. of green drink powder. Make this in a juicer fresh by adding 2 zuchini. 1 handful of dandelion leaves, 1 potato and 1 apple. If you need more to make a cup of juice add more dandelion leaves and zuchini and another apple if you need it to taste better. You can have a couple cups of this before lunch if you want. This can be Kyo-green, Barleygreen, Green Magma, Spirulina, Barley Juice Powder or Wheat Grass Powder or simply make the carrot juice and eat a couple handfuls of fresh sprouts with it.
- Lunch
  - Have a BIG salad of raw vegetables either as a salad or as simply cut up raw veggies. Buy a variety of vegetables and make different combinations each day.
  - 1 portion of grain, no wheat allowed
  - Have a vegetable main dish
  - Ideas: Vegetable stir fry with oriental spices, Italian spices, Greek, Mexican or Middle Eastern
  - Spices, you can also bake your vegetables in a sauce with the spices mentioned. You are allowed to use 1 tsp. of oil per meal and a little salt. You will make your life easier if you can follow the general formulas on the next page.
- Repeat morning snack.
- Dinner is the same as lunch but without grain.

General Rules

- You are allowed 1 serving of grain a day at lunch.
- You are allowed unlimited vegetables. You should try to cook them a little since your condition will not tolerate a lot of raw vegetables.
- You are allowed up to three fruits as a snack.
- You are allowed only fresh juices or vegetables for your snack.
- You must drink the juice with green powder. This is what will keep you full.
- There is no meat or milk products or eggs or fish allowed on this diet.
- There are of course no packaged goods, sugars, colas, sodas or coffee or tea allowed either.

Must

- Walk every day to sweat or at least every other day. Since you do not walk now start out small. Just get in the HABIT by walking around the block every night for a while. Then work up from there.
- Shower or bathe daily with loufa Drink lots of water. 10 glasses a day is ideal for your weight. More is better too!

General Formula for Cooking Interesting Vegetable Dishes

Dr. John McDougall has the best cookbooks for vegan cooking and just came out with one on how to make meals in 10 minutes or less. His cookbooks are the best but here are some simple formulas you can follow too. You only need any combination of fresh and frozen vegetables you have around that seem to go together, a cooking method, and a spice theme. You can add up to 2 TBS. of nuts and/or raisins (sultanas) to your dishes to make them more interesting.

Stir Fry
- 1 tsp. of oil
- 1/2 tsp. of salt
- 1 onion and some garlic
- Sauté these in the oil and then add the spice mix for your "national flavor."
- Add vegetables and sauté until cooked but not wilted.

Baked Vegetables
- 1 tsp. of oil
- 1/2 tsp. of salt
- onion and garlic
- Sauté the above
- Add the vegetables and 2-3 cups of vegetable stock and spices
- Bake for 1 hour in a covered dish
- When finished pour off the liquid into a sauce pan
- Add a little cornstarch with cold water to the sauce pan to make a thick "gravy" for the veggies.

Stuffed Veggies
Use any of the leftovers from the methods above to stuff baked squash, potatoes, or yams. You can also steam green peppers or tomatoes and stuff those.

My Favorite Combinations
- Broccoli, cauliflower and red pepper with Italian seasoning
- Zucchini, tomato, peppers, green beans, eggplant and mushrooms with Italian seasoning
- Zucchini, corn, tomato, mushrooms, pimentos, red peppers, green peppers and yellow peppers with Mexican seasoning
- Baby corn, peas (snow peas if you can find), mushrooms, greens, sprouts, broccoli, peppers, and carrots with Oriental seasoning
- Green peppers, celery, onions, greens, walnuts and raisins stuffed in squash. Peas and carrots in tomato sauce with Middle Eastern seasoning. You can think of anything from here! Serve vegetables over baked potatoes, mashed potatoes, grated potatoes, squash or grated zucchini instead of grain.

Salad Ideas
- Swiss chard, arugula and lettuce chopped up with mushrooms, tomatoes, cucumbers
- Grated red and green cabbage and carrots mixed with any salad
- Chopped up broccoli, cauliflower, carrots, red peppers, green peppers, yellow peppers, spring onions, sprouts, etc.

Spice Mixtures for Vegetables

Barbecue Seasoning
- 4 TBS. paprika
- 2 TBS. each garlic and onion powder
- 2 tsp. each dry mustard and ground thyme
- 1 tsp. black pepper
- 1/2 tsp. cayenne

Cajun Blackened Seasoning
- 2 tsp. paprika
- 1 tsp. each black pepper, basil, cumin seed, caraway, fennel, thyme, oregano and white pepper
- 1/2 tsp. each crushed red pepper, salt

Chinese Five Spices
- 1 TBS. each cinnamon, star anise (ground)
- 1/2 tsp. each (ground) fennel, black pepper, cloves
- Chili Powder
- 3 TBS. paprika
- 2 TBS. cumin
- 1 TBS. each turmeric, garlic, cayenne and salt

Curry Powder
- 2 TBS. coriander
- 2 TBS. fenugreek
- 1/2 tsp. cumin
- 1/2 tsp. white pepper
- 1/2 tsp. ginger
- 1 1/2 TBS. cayenne (or too taste) Grind in grinder until powder

Curry Powder #2
- 6 TBS. coriander
- 1 TBS. each turmeric, fenugreek, and cumin
- 1/2 TBS. cardamom
- 1/2 tsp. ground cloves
- 1/8 tsp. cayenne

Greek Seasoning
- 2 TBS. each onion powder, paprika, black pepper, oregano, and bell pepper
- 1 TBS. Basil
- 2 tsp. lemon thyme (or lemon zest)
- Grind to a powder

Italian Seasoning: Fresh
- 1/2 cup each: parsley, basil, marjoram
- 1/4 cup each thyme and rosemary

Italian Season: Dried
- 2 TBS. each oregano, marjoram, thyme, basil leaves
- 1 TBS. each rosemary and sage

Mexican Seasoning
- 2 TBS. Chili pepper, crushed
- 1 TBS. each: garlic powder, onion, paprika, oregano
- 2 tsp. each cumin, celery seed and cayenne
- 1 tsp. ground bay leaf

Persian Seasoning: Fresh
- 1/2 cup parsley and coriander and chives
- 1/4 cup mint
- Add this fresh mix to any dish

Egyptian Seasoning
- 2 tsp. coriander
- 1 TBS. cumin
- 1/2 tsp. allspice
- 1 tsp. garlic powder

Anti-Hypoglycemia Diet

Daily Schedule
- Breakfast
  - Green omelet with tea and oatmeal (plain or with raisins and apple)
  - Cottage cheese and fruit with plain oatmeal
  - Yogurt and Muesli (dry oats, raisins and walnuts is a simple homemade muesli)
- Lunch and Dinner
  - Beef kebab made with beef, chopped fresh herbs, rice or oatmeal, an egg and some shredded veggies. Vegetable side dish. Cucumber/yogurt salad
  - Mexican beans and rice. Stir fry chopped fresh parsley and coriander and onion and garlic in a little olive oil. Add rice and beans (already cooked) and frozen green beans and spices and salt. Heat through. Serve with fresh argula (jarjir) or chard.
  - Tabouli with NO burghl. Make with a little feta cheese instead. Serve with "Turkish Rice": Sauté onions, celery, chopped fresh coriander and parsley and garlic and green peppers in olive oil. Add ground beef. Pour this sauté over the rice.
  - White tuna with rice. Stir fry celery, green pepper, onion and garlic in a little olive oil. Add cooked rice. Put one can of white tuna over the top. Eat with fresh greens (chard and jarjir).
  - Lamb or chicken kebab (make the same as number one only use ground lamb or chicken). Serve with yogurt sauce and fresh greens. Yogurt sauce: Take one carton of yogurt , add to it 1 tsp. turmeric, 1 tsp. coriander, 1/2 tsp. salt. Fry some onion and garlic in a little ghee. Add the yogurt to this sauté and stir quickly, Serve as a side "dip" for the kufta. Serve with fresh greens.
  - Stir fry. Use at least half fresh vegetables (you can use some frozen as well), stir fry with olive oil, garlic, onion and freshly grated ginger and 1 tsp. allspice. Sauté meat first, then vegetables. Use tuna or stew beef chopped small or chicken breast. Serve over plain rice.
- Snacks

  - Homemade humus with vegetables to dip: celery, carrots, apple, green pepper
  - Pumpkin seeds and raisins
  - Apples and sunflower seeds
  - Broccoli and slice of cheese
  - Smoked salmon, tomato and Swiss chard and a piece of bread
  - Avocado and tomato on pita bread

General Rules
- Do not serve leftovers as a meal. You can use leftovers to cook with but not as a meal. Examples: Use leftover stir fry and grind the veggies up in the kufta, use leftover kufta to put over "Turkish Rice", use leftover rice to cook in Mexican rice dish or in kufta, etc...So you can USE the leftovers to cook with but

- NEVER re-heat things as a meal.
- Every meal must have a salad. Keep the salads simple. No tomato, no lettuce. Serve cucumber yogurt salad, tabouli without burghul or just simply wash some jarjir and chard and put it on a plate.
- Do not skip an mealtimes
    - 8:00 AM
    - 10:30 snack
    - 12:00 PM
    - 3:00 snack
    - 5:00 PM
    - 8-9:00 snack
- Take Tea 30 minutes before meal (if hcp give you or if you want)
- Take any vitamins or supplements with meal
- The keys are
    - Planning, you must always have enough food in the house and prepared for EACH meal
    - Snack before they get hungry. If hypoglycemic is allowed to wait for a meal or get very hungry this will set off temper outbursts, low blood sugar attacks, pain attacks, fainting, dizziness and nausea. Whoever is cooking - you need to have the food ready on schedule and on time.
    - Do not wait get hungry for a meal. Make the meals on time and eat at least a little.

Foods to Avoid
- Sugar
- Coffee or tea or sodas (or any caffeine)
- Chocolate
- Milk or wheat (alone or in great quantity)
- Packaged goods (even if they say they are healthy)
- Sugar substitutes
- Processed foods
- Pasta
- Fast Foods
- Pastries, cakes, cookies or roll

Shopping List
Check the house daily. Make sure you are well stocked in all of these things. If you plan well, you should be shopping only once a week. Get things replenished as soon as they run out!
- To buy in bulk then freeze/store
    - Ground Beef Ground Lamb Chicken Breast
    - White Tuna (canned) Smoked Salmon (optional)
    - Stewing Beef
    - Brown Rice
    - Brown Basmati Rice
    - Oatmeal
    - Muesli

- Spices
- Salt (sea salt ONLY) Frozen spinach
- Frozen green beans
- Feta Cheese (boxes of) Raisins
- Pumpkin seeds
- Garbanzo (humus beans) Tahini
- Olive oil
- To buy from veggie market or supermarket
  - Avocado (optional)
  - Parsley potatoes
  - Onions
  - Garlic coriander jarjir
  - Swiss chard
  - Green peppers (red, orange, yellow OK too)
  - Green beans (when in season)
  - Broccoli cauliflower lemons limes carrots
  - Apples (not green, only red varieties)
  - Mung bean or alfalfa sprouts for stir fry
  - Fresh dill for kufta and cucumber yogurt salad
  - Allowed fruits like: apricot, peaches, plums, guava, mango, banana, pears, apples
- To buy from the supermarket when needed
  - Yogurt
  - Cottage cheese
  - Cheddar cheese

The Haas Detox

This is the best detox I have found for congested conditions. I have about ten detoxes that I share with students and have used all of them myself at least once too.

Daily Schedule
- Pre-Breakfast, after waking up
  - Drink two glasses of water, one glass with half a lemon squeezed into it
  - Drink any herbal tea you have at this time
- Breakfast
  - Eat a couple pieces of raw fruit, chewing well to mix with your saliva.
  - Take any vitamins you have at this time.
  - After you FINISH the fruit, start making your grain. Make yourself either a bowl of rice, a bowl of oatmeal or a bowl of barley. You may put TWO TBS. of molasses or honey on your grain to sweeten it or eat it made in stock with salt as a savory grain.
- Lunch, noon to 1pm, make yourself 1-2 bowls of steamed vegetables or stir fried in a little water with garlic, onion and a little salt and spices. You can use up to 1 tsp. of olive oil.
- Snack, you may only drink vegetable juices for a snack. Preferably this is the juice from the vegetables you have been cooking that you saved. You can also make carrot celery juice if you wish. Drink your herbal tea at this time. You may eat raw vegetables if you need.
- Dinner, from 5pm to 6 pm, same as lunch but take your vitamins again here.
- Night, drink your herbal tea at this time again. Do not eat any more food.

Foods to Avoid
- Oil
- Salt
- MSG
- Milk
- Tea
- Candy
- Snacks
- Bread
- Sugar
- Honey

Do not use Chicken bouillon cubes to cook with during this time. Use only fresh vegetable broth, water or homemade chicken broth.

Ideas

- Stir Fry vegetables
- Chop veggies in a pot and bake them in a tomato or other sauce for 30 minute in a covered pan
- Use oatmeal to thicken soups and sauces, then blend some in the blender for a creamy soup.
- Slice vegetables in fingers and steam or bake with curry powder or fresh herbs
- Zucchini and carrots with fresh dill
- Potatoes with chives, garlic and onions
- Potatoes with fresh dill and a bit of mustard
- Bisilla, bemia, fusulia all made without oil and no rice
- Soups
- Oatmeal - plain (for kids with apple and raisin)
- Raw vegetables cut up
- Chopped salads with lettuce, tomato, onion, broccoli, cauliflower, peppers, and carrots.
- Zucchini and tomato stir fry with chopped spinach or parsley and Italian season
- Tomato Soup with green pepper, carrot and squash
- Broccoli and cauliflower stir fry

Tips

- Chop up carrots, celery, broccoli, cauliflower, etc. and keep them in a container for when anyone gets hungry. Keep a basket of apples and oranges out for the children when they get hungry. Use any leftover stir fries for soups the next day. Use a lot of fresh herbs or spices to make up for the lack of salt. Make a glass of carrot or carrot celery juice for a snack. (You can add an apple to the juice to make it sweeter but it must all be homemade juice).
- Make it simple! Make oatmeal for breakfast with mint tea and then soup and salad for lunch. When you are stuck make soup or raw veggies. Buy some frozen peas & carrots, and canned beets and green beans for quick snacks-emergency hunger.
- Preplan your meals and think about what you will make all week before you start. This will make shopping and cooking easier to plan. Don't worry about making the same thing more than once.
- Drink a lot of water.
- Plan to eat a small nibble of veggies, glass of carrot juice or apple between the meals so you will not be hungry. Plan ahead! Perhaps prepare some meals, shop and plan for two days before you start.

Must

- Walk every day to sweat.
- Shower or bathe daily with loufa.
- Drink lots of water. 8-10 glasses.

Low Carbohydrate Diet

(Not a protein diet or overly high in protein)

- Meals
    - Breakfast: "Protein" drink or meal.
    - Lunch: "Protein" meal
    - Evening: Starch meal
    - Snacks: Must include a vegetable with a small portion of carbohydrate, starch and/or protein
    - Last meal of the day: Note that if you have been "good" all day your body should feel balanced and you can probably afford to have one of your favorite foods with or as a "desert" with dinner. Test this out. As long as adding favorite foods does not interfere with your sleep it should be fine to do at this last meal of the day in moderation of course!

Daily Schedule
- Breakfast
    - Scrambled Tofu* or Scrambled Eggs with sliced tomato and cucumbers on the side
    - Soy Milk Shake (recipe on your original printout)
    - Smoked Salmon with onion served on romaine lettuce instead of bread
    - Tuna with green pepper and onion and tomato chopped up into a "salad"
    - No STARCHES ALLOWED! No bread, rice, potatoes or anything starchy.
- Snacks
    - When you get hungry drink one of the snacks I recommended on your original printout.
    - Use fenugreek tea (helba) and the energy drinks.
    - Drink freshly made carrot celery juice or freshly cut up raw vegetables.
    - Never have any carbohydrates as snacks. Only at the last meal of the day.
- Protein Meals, any vegetable combination with any meat or protein like beans, tofu, eggs, cheese or nuts. Do not each starchy vegetables for this meal like potatoes, yams, peas, corn, and squash
    - Vegetable salad (dark greens of any kind including broccoli, green peppers and green leafy vegetables) along with any other fresh vegetables you like.
    - Protein of some sort: fish, cheese, tofu, meat, eggs. Do not eat lunch meat or fried or breaded meats.
    - Vegetable side dish like stir fry vegetables or baked vegetables or even plain cooked green beans with mushroom sauce or broccoli with lemon and pepper.
- Starch Meals, any vegetable combination with rice or oatmeal or barley.
    - Vegetable salad with DARK GREENS like spinach, argula and chard along with other fresh vegetables or tabouli.
    - Stir fry vegetables or baked vegetables
    - Rice, barley or oatmeal, potatoes, yams, squash or whole grain bread.
    - Try to avoid breads as much as you can but you can use whole wheat pita

occasionally if needed and any bread in a situation when you just can't find anything else.

*Scrambled Tofu: Mock Scrambled Eggs

- Ingredients
    - 1 box tofu, drained
    - 1/8 t.turmeric (more or less according to taste)
    - 1 t. Mckays chicken style seasoning (or salt to taste)
    - 2 T. oil
    - 1/2 lb. fresh mushrooms chopped (optional)
    - 1 green onion, chopped fine (optional)
    - 1/2 t. garlic powder
    - 1 bell pepper, chopped fine (optional)
- Directions
    - Place tofu in hot skillet, breaking up with fork or spatula into chunks. Add to chopped tofu the remaining ingredients. Cook until well mixed and liquid is gone.
    - Serves: 4-6
    - Preparation time: 15 mins

Food to Avoid
- Sugar
- White Flour
- Packaged or canned foods (frozen is OK)
- Breads
- Sodas
- Synthetic or restaurant foods

The Non-Toxic Diet

The following guidelines will help you plan a healthy eating style for your family. Keep in mind that it is hard for anyone to achieve perfection all of the time. Try to strive to this model but don't create too much stress trying to achieve it. Give yourself time to get used to it and room to make mistakes. Sometimes it takes a few years before healthy eating is truly second nature!

- Eat Organic if you can
- Drink filtered water
- Rotate your foods (especially common allergens like milk, milk products, eggs, wheat, and yeast foods)
- Practice food combining
- Eat natural, seasonal cuisine native to the region
- Use as much as you can from this list:
    - Fruits
    - Vegetables
    - whole grains
    - legumes, nuts
    - seeds
    - fresh fish
    - poultry
- Cook in stainless steel, iron, glass or porcelain or clay. Do not use aluminum.
- Avoid or minimize: red meats, cured meats, organ meats, refined foods, canned foods, sugar, salt, saturated fats, coffee, tea, alcohol and nicotine.

You must strike a balance between a healthy rotation diet and a stress-free life. If you create a rotation that is too difficult and causes much stress you may cancel out any benefit you gain from it. So start with what you know you can do and increase the difficulty **OR** start with the most difficult diet and give yourself permission to add to it if you need to! And if at any time you feel the need just give yourself a break of a few days and then start again.

Create Your Own Diet

First, look at the food list below. Cross out anything you know you are allergic too (and its family members. Note that peanuts are a member of the legume family so if you are allergic to peanuts you are allergic to legumes!). If you want to really take this to the ultimate effect, also cross out anything that you eat often and try to also eliminate those things for the first six weeks of your rotation. Then gradually introduce them. Next, select a carbohydrate for each day of the diet. Begin with complex carbohydrates; select the following complex carbohydrates - white sweet potato, water chestnut, malanga, arrow-root, yam (true yam from family Dioscore-aceae), lotus, cassava All of these complex carbohydrates are gluten-free. Eliminate any food from the above list that you have eaten frequently or that you know causes symptoms.

If you have severe allergies don't include any member of the grass family in your diet - wheat, corn, oats, rice, rye, barley, millet, spelt, teff, milo. This is the most common group of problem foods in the plant kingdom. Do not include commonly eaten complex carbohydrates such as potatoes initially in the diet. Do not include any members of the legume family initially in the diet. Do not include any seed- based complex carbohydrates such as amaranth, buckwheat, and beans initially in the diet. Also, select some vegetables for each day of the diet elect a meat for each day of the diet - do not initially include eggs, chicken, bovine, or milks and milk products from the bovine family. Select an oil/nut for each day (not nuts if candida or mold sensitive) and select a fruit for each day (if no candida or mold sensitivities.)

To make a regular rotation diet simply make a chart following the instructions above and rotate food groups every four-seven days making sure to eliminate food groups you know you are allergic too (if you are allergic to one food in the group you are allergic to the rest as well). After 6 weeks re-introduce foods and gauge reactions.

For a diagnosis and allergy cure diet post this diet and make very simple menu plans for the foods listed. You should be eating very simple, nothing fancy, very easy and you should be eating as if you are "breathing" or drinking water. Don't expect it to be anexciting experience. Find something else to excite you the next few weeks. (Although trying new foods is exciting to some people). Stick to this diet for 4 weeks keeping a daily record of how you feel and any allergic reactions you may have. On week 5 eliminate any foods which have caused you a reaction the past four weeks and re-introduce food groups that you have not tried or that you are least likely to react to. Introduce a new food group every four days. Cross the group out if you see a reaction. Remember you are staying with your original rotation and simply ADDING to the list you already have a new food group every four days. After a few more weeks of adding new food groups every day and eliminating the ones you reacted to and the previously crossed out ones, you should now have an expanded rotation diet for yourself. When you reach this "expanded rotation diet" and have no food groups left to test then Follow this for 4 weeks. After 4 weeks start introducing all previously crossed out groups to see if any reaction is still there. Continue to keep away from any items that still cause reaction. Stick to your (constantly revised) program and re-check allergic items every 6 weeks. Within six months you should have nothing crossed out.

The ideal diet is a seven to ten day rotation, but this is very difficult, so start out with a four day rotation.

- Greens, veggies, and Herbs
    - Algae: Agar-Agar, carrageen, kelp (kombu)
    - Chenopodiiaceae: Beet, chard, lamb's quarters, spinach, sugar beet
    - Compositae: Artichoke, chamomile, chicory, dandelion, endive, escarole, lettuce, safflower, sunflower seeds, tarragon.
    - Cruciferae: Horseradish, mustard, rashish, rutabaga, turnip, watercress, cabbage, broccoli, Brussels sprouts, cabbage kraut, cauliflower, Chinese cabbage, collards, kale, kohlrabi
    - Discoreaceae: Chinese potato and yam
    - Iridaceae: Saffron
    - Lauraceae: Avocado, bay leaf, cinnamon, sassafrass
    - Labiatae: Basil, catnip, horehound, lemon balm, marjoram, mint, oregano, peppermint, rosemary, sage, savory, spearmint, thyme
    - Liliacea: Asparagus, chive, garlic, leek, onion, sarsaparilla, shallot
    - Malvaceae: Cottonseed, hibiscus, okra, jute
    - Myraceae: Allspice, clove, guava
    - Nightshade: Eggplant, potato, tobacco, tomato, all peppers, paprika, pimento, cayenne
    - Papaveraceae: Poppy seed
    - Portulacaceae: Purslane
    - Umbelliferae: Carrot, ceriac, celery, lovage, parsley, parsnip, angelica, anise, caraway, celery seeds, coriander, cumin, dill, fennel
    - Zingiberacea: Cardamom, ginger, turmeric

- Meats
    - Bovine: Beef, veal, buffalo, goat, sheep, lamb, mutton, milk from and milk products from
    - Camel: Camel and llama
    - Deer: Deer, venison, elk, moose, reindeer
    - Hare: Hare and rabbit
    - Dove: Dove and pidgeon
    - Duck: Duck, goose and eggs from
    - Grouse: Partridge
    - Pheasant: Chicken, Cornish hen, seafowel, pheasant, quail and eggs from
    - Turkey: Turkey and their eggs'

- Fish
    - Anchovy: Anchovy
    - Bass: White Perch and yellow bass
    - Bluefish: bluefish
    - Catfish: Catfish
    - Codfish: Cod, scrod, cusk, haddock, pollack, whitng
    - Croaker (saltwater): Croaker, drum, sea trout, silver perch, spot weakfish, spotted sea trout

- o Eel: American eel
- o Flounder: Dab, flounder, halibut, plaice, sole, turbout
- o Harvestfish: Butterfish, harvestfish
- o Herring: Shad
- o Herring (saltwater): Pilchard, sea herring
- o Jack: Amberjack, pompano, yellow jack
- o Mackerel: Albacore, bonito, mackerel, tuna
- o Minnow: Carp, chub
- o Perch: Sauger, walleye, yellow perch
- o Pike: Muskellunge, pickerel, pike
- o Salmon: All salmon and trout
- o Swordfish: Swordfish
- o Whitefish: whitefish

- **Shellfish**
  - o Clam: Clam
  - o Cockle: Cockle
  - o Crab: Crab
  - o Lobster: Crayfish, langostinos, lobster
  - o Oyster: Oyster
  - o Scallop: Scallop
  - o Shrimp: Prawns, shrimp
  - o Snail: Snail

- **Oils and Nuts**
  - o Anacardiaceae: Cashew, mango, pistachio
  - o Coniferae: Juniper berries, pine nuts
  - o Cruciferae: Canola oil
  - o Fagaceae: Beechnut and chestnut
  - o Betulaceae: Filbert, hazelnut, oil of birch (wintergreen)
  - o Juglandaceae: Black walnut, butternut, English walnut, hickory nut, pecan
  - o Laurel: Avocado oil, avocados
  - o Lecythidaceae: Brazil nut
  - o Linaceae: Flaxseeds, flax seed oil
  - o Oleaceae: Olives, olive oil
  - o Palmacea: Coconut oil
  - o Pedaliaceae: Sesame seed
  - o Protea: Macadamia nuts

- **Grains and Carbs**
  - o Goosefoot: Amaranth, Quinoa
  - o Convolvulaceae: Jicama, sweet potato
  - o Cyperaceae: Chinese water chestnuts
  - o Leguminosae: Alfalfa, bean (kidney, lentil, lima, mung, navy, pinto, soy, string), carob, guar gum, gum acacia, kudzu, licorice, pea (black-eyed, chick-pea, green), peanut

- Marantacea: Arrowroot
- Polygonaceae: Buckwheat, garden sorrel, rhubarb
- Gramineae: Bamboo shoots, barley, corn, lemongrass, millet, oats, rice, rye, sorghum, sugarcane, wheat, wild rice

- **Fruits**
  - Actinidiaceae: Kiwi fruit
  - Annonaceae: custard-apple, pawpaw, cherimoya
  - Bromeliaceae: Pinneapple
  - Caprifoliaceae: Honeysuckle, elderberry
  - Caricaceae: Papaya
  - Cucurbitacea: Cantaloupe, cucumber, gherkin, honeydew, muskmelon, pumpkin, squash, watermelon
  - Ebonaceae: Persimmon
  - Ericaceae: Blueberry, cranberry, huckleberry
  - Moracea: Breadfruit, fig, mulberry
  - Punicacea: Pomegranete
  - Rosaceae: Apple, blackberry, boysenberry, dewberry, loganberry, raspberry, rose hips, strawberry
  - Musaceae: Banana and plantain
  - Rutaceae: Citron, grapefruit, kumquat, lemon, lime, orange, pomelo, tangelo, tangerine, citrus, rue
  - Saxifragacea: Currant, gooseberry
  - Vitacea: Grape

- **Other**
  - Aceraceae: Maple Syrup
  - Euphorbiaceae: Tapioca
  - Orchidadea: Vanilla
  - Palmaceae: Coconut, date, sago palm starch
  - Sterculiaceae: Chocolate, cocoa, cola, gum karaya
  - Theacea: Tea
  - Fungi: Mold in cheeses, mushroom, truffle, yeast
  - Honey

For People with Candida, Very Severe Allergies, Eczema, or Asthma

Do not include any member of the grass family in your diet - wheat, corn, oats, rice, rye, barley, millet, spelt, teff, milo. This is the most common group of problem foods in the plant kingdom.

Do not include any member of the bovid family either; this is the number one problem food family in the animal kingdom. The bovid family includes beef, goats, buffalo, lamb and sheep. Do not include milk or any dairy products. Do not include any other commonly eaten meats such as chicken and pork.

If you are, or your child is, very sensitive to mold, do not include nuts in the diet. Do not include any fruit that you either know or think you might react to either. If you are very mold sensitive, do not include fruit in the diet. You are not allowed any sugar, coffee, sodas, refined or processed foods, packaged foods, canned foods. All foods must be fresh or frozen. These items should NEVER be part of your diet.

During this diet you will become extra sensitive and start to notice all your allergies more. So try to use unscented soaps in the bath and for your clothes washing, use sea salt to brush your teeth (or very plain toothpaste), don't clean or use commercial cleaners (baking soda and vinegar are fine), and try to stay away from perfumes and deodorants and chemicals. Keep in mind there are other factors that will aggravate your allergies. Eczema is aggravated by the sun, asthma by heavy exercise and stress and most all allergies by stress, lack of sleep, arguing, etc...Get enough sleep, relax and get moderate sun.

Drink only spring or filtered water, remember to rotate herbs and spices, and do not "cheat" or do a "partial diet". This will be ineffective and will not work. Do it right or don't do it at all. On the 2-4th day of the start of the diet (the bare-bones-nothing-allergic-plan) you will notice a worsening of your symptoms as the last residues of your allergic foods detox out. So if you have eczema you will get a flare up of it on the 2-4th day of an elimination/rotation diet, etc.

Universal Parasite Cleanse

Note you must take the remedies for ten days on then five days off in at least three cycles and up to ten cycles to take care of all un-hatched eggs that may still be in your body. Italics indicates this is safe for kids.

1. Cleanse the colon with food and laxative herbs.
    a. Eat 1/4 to 1/3 cup of raw rice for breakfast, chewing well and do not eat again for three hours.
    b. Take Cascara Sagrada (with red raspberry and fennel and/or licorice) at night time (1-2 tsp. per cup of water. Make as a decoction).
    c. *Eat dried figs, prunes or drink prune juice*
    d. Drink dandelion root tea (make as a decoction 1-2 tsp. of root per cup of water)
    e. *Drink Turkey Rhubarb Tea (same directions as above).*

2. Take a nutritional tea or supplement three times a day.
    a. Alfalfa, *licorice*, dandelion, *marshmallow, rose hips*, nettles, *oat straw, red raspberry.* Mix all the above herbs together in a tea or mix and match. Make as an infusion. 1-2 tsp. of herb per cup of water)
    b. or take a natural green supplement like Barleygreen or Kyogreen or Juice Plus

3. Take a vermifuge or vermicide herb to kill and expel the parasites.
    a. Black walnut - 1 tsp. powder daily or 2 OO capsules daily (each capsule has 1/2 tsp. of powder). and one of the below or a combination of the below assorted:
    b. Wormwood or wormseed (potentially toxic) 25 drops or two capsules 30 minutes before each meal (dosage same for all below for adults).
    c. *Turkey Rhubarb (safe for kids)*
    d. *Thyme*
    e. *Fennel*
    f. *Sage*
    g. Colloidal silver (for weak people)
    h. Citrus Seed extract - 3 drops one time daily.
    i. Aloe Vera Juice - 1-3 oz. 1 or two times daily.
    j. Mugwort tea
    k. Take betel nut powder 30 grams before breakfast *(5-10 grams for kids)*. Worms should expel in 9 hours or less.
    l. If your system can stand it take 3 cloves of RAW garlic 3-5 times a day in salad, or plain. For kids use 1 cloves three times a day. You can slice it and put it between apple slices to cut the bite of the garlic. Tastes great!

4. Take Substance to absorb the toxins that are released.
    a. Betonite clay
    b. Raw potato juice - 1/2 cup to 1 cup daily.
    c. Fresh raw apple juice - 2-3 cups daily

5. Take an herb to create bulk and push toxins out.
    a. Psyllium husk powder (if stuck for sources you can use Metamucil). Take two heaping tsp. in a glass of juice or water twice a day.
    b. Flax seeds - same dosage as above.
    c. Make fenugreek tea and drink the seeds with the tea.

6. Replenish the friendly bacteria in your colon.
    a. Rejuvalac
    b. Oat Yogurt
    c. Raw, saltless sauerkraut (homemade)
    d. Acidophilis tablets
    e. Sesame seed yogurt

7. Replenish your body with electrolytes and enzymes.
    a. Fresh juices like carrot, celery and beet (dried beet is best)
    b. Readymade electrolyte blend or mineral blend
    c. Eat raw pineapple and figs

8. Follow a fasting diet plan.
    a. Anti-acid diet (Hay diet) with no meat, only vegetable protein.
    b. Haas Detox
    c. Juice Fast
    d. Unani Tibb Detox without meat
    e. Also: try to avoid raw foods and parasitic produce and concentrate on anti-parasite foods like: beet, cabbage, carrot, garlic, leek, onion, radish, fennel, cloves, cayenne, pumpkin seeds (raw), ginger, sage, and thyme.

9. Take anti-oxidants.
    a. Milk thistle, zinc, vitamin B, Gingko, C, E, B6, Etc...
    b. A readymade anti-oxidant formula
    c. If you are using the herbal teas above (in B) you probably don't need this.
    d. Make fresh juices (carrot-celery, etc...) daily and drink at least 3-4 cups a day.

High-Phosphorus: Alkaline Diet

- Epsom Salt Bath twice a week.
- The only oil to be used is olive oil in small quantities
- Use minimal salt
- Meals
    - Pre-Breakfast: lemon water every day
    - Breakfast: Fruit only
    - Lunch: Starch meal
    - Evening: Protein meal
    - Snacks: vegetables only or freshly made juices, trail mix
    - Trail Mix: Brazil Nuts, Almonds, Raisins, Sunflower Seeds, Pumkin Seeds

Daily Schedule
- Breakfast
    - Saturday: orange and grapefruit with dates
    - Sunday: orange and pineapple with dates
    - Monday: apples and banana with figs
    - Tuesday: dark grapes and apricots
    - Wednesday: figs, dates, dark grapes and red apples
    - Thursday: Black currants or raisins with apples
    - Friday: pomegranate and banana with raisins or figs or dates
- Starch Meals, any vegetable combination with any grain (except wheat) like:
    - Monday: veggie with brown rice
    - Tuesday: veggie with barley
    - Wednesday: veggie with oatmeal
    - Thursday: veggie with brown rice
    - Friday: veggie with barley
    - Saturday: veggie with brown rice
    - Sunday: veggie with oatmeal
- Protein Meals, any vegetable combination with a meat. You are only allowed ONE PROTEIN A MEAL, you cannot combine yogurt with meat or buts with tofu or anything like that. Here are the specific proteins I recommend each day since I also recommend you avoid for now much red meat or chicken and also milk and milk products:
    - Monday: poached eggs
    - Tuesday: liver
    - Wednesday: garbanzo soup/stew
    - Thursday: fish
    - Friday: poached eggs
    - Saturday: *green lentil soup
    - Sunday: Goats cheese or goats milk

*Green Lentil Soup
- Stir fry fresh chopped onion and garlic in olive oil.
- Add 1 cup of orange lentils and 1/4 cup rice and three cups of chicken or vegetable stock or salted water.
- Simmer until soup consitency
- Add 1-2 cups chopped greens.
- Simmer one half hour more

General Rules

- Begin each meal with a raw food (vegetable salad) made from dark greens with shredded carrots.
- Eat fruit separate from other things and do not combine with other foods or meals
- Do not drink water or other drinks with the meal. Do not drink milk or eat cheese.
- Do not eat proteins and starches together (bread and meat or bread with cheese or baked potato with meat) EVER!
-

Give yourself three days to one week to adapt and then continue for three weeks on this "diet". The only thing this diet eliminates is processed foods, unnatural fats and oils, sugar and pure milk. It allows you all other foods within limits so you are not being deprived, you are simply limiting and re-proportioning for a while.

Foods to Avoid
- Coffee
- Sugar
- White Flour
- Packaged or canned foods (frozen is OK)
- Tea with Caffeine
- Sodas
- Synthetic or restaurant foods

Kidney and Lung: Alkaline Diet

- Meals
  - Breakfast: Fruit only
  - Lunch: Starch meal
  - Evening: Protein meal
  - Snacks: vegetables only or freshly made juices, trail mix, black sesame seeds, walnuts

Daily Schedule
- Breakfast
  - Saturday: apples with dates
  - Sunday: mandarin orange and pineapple with dates
  - Monday: apples and banana with figs
  - Tuesday: mangos and apricots
  - Wednesday: watermelon and star fruit
  - Thursday: Black currants or raisins with apples
  - Friday: pomegranate and pears and figs
- Starch Meals, any vegetable combination with any grain (except wheat) like the ones listed below. Emphasize the vegetables: Spinach, green string beans, any DARK GREENS!
  - Monday: veggie with brown rice
  - Tuesday: veggie with barley
  - Wednesday: veggie with yams
  - Thursday: veggie with brown rice
  - Friday: veggie with barley
  - Saturday: veggie with brown rice
  - Sunday: veggie with oatmeal
- Protein Meals, any vegetable combination with a meat. You are only allowed ONE PROTEIN A MEAL, you cannot combine yogurt with meat or buts with tofu or anything like that. Here are the specific proteins I recommend each day since I also recommend you avoid for now much red meat or chicken and also milk and milk products:
  - Monday: tofu
  - Tuesday: kidney
  - Wednesday: eggs
  - Thursday: kidney beans
  - Friday: shrimp
  - Saturday: chicken liver
  - Sunday: Goats cheese or goats milk

General Rules

- Begin each meal with a raw food (vegetable salad) made from dark greens with shredded carrots.
- Eat fruit separate from other things and do not combine with other foods or meals
- Do not drink water or other drinks with the meal
- Do not drink milk or eat cheese.
- Do not eat proteins and starches together (bread and meat or bread with cheese or baked potato with meat) EVER!
-

Give yourself three days to one week to adapt and then continue for three weeks on this "diet". The only thing this diet eliminates is processed foods, unnatural fats and oils, sugar and pure milk. It allows you all other foods within limits so you are not being deprived, you are simply limiting and re-proportioning for a while.

Foods to Avoid
- Coffee
- Sugar
- White Flour
- Packaged or canned foods (frozen is OK)
- Tea with Caffeine
- Sodas
- Synthetic or restaurant foods

~Section Five: Supplements~

Nutritional Healing with Supplements: Is it Possible?
By Kristie Burns, Mh, ND

With calcium being added to orange juice and multivitamins to bread and cereals, it is difficult to escape supplements. However, this relatively new addition to our diet is not as necessary and healthy as advertisements proclaim. If supplements are not used with the same care and supervision as prescription drugs they can be harmful. Used as dietary tools, these processed supplements can never provide people with the nutrition that they need.

Supplemental nutrition is not to be confused with the true value of a balanced diet, however. Nutritional awareness is an important part of planning one's daily menu. In fact, the value of certain foods in maintaining health was recognized long before the first vitamins were actually identified. In the 18th century, for example it was demonstrated that the addition of citrus fruits to the diet would prevent the development of scurvy. However, the idea of creating scientifically measured and condensed pill-like nutritional substitutes and supplements to food has only been around since the early 1900's and is one of modern medicine's largest human experiments (Cybernorth).

Supplements can never truly provide people with the nutrients they need. First of all, supplement information is often measured on an inaccurate scale. The US RDA's are based on the amount of vitamins one needs to consume each day to keep a normal healthy male from getting any deficiency disease such as scurvy. The US RDA's do not indicate how much of a vitamin a person needs for optimum health and they do not take into consideration other factors such as pregnancy, nursing, illness, inherited vitamin deficiencies, environment or age (Balch). Secondly, foods contain an endless amount of nutrients of various kinds, which have yet to be truly duplicated. Apples alone contain more than 450 identified phytochemicals, some having been identified only in the past ten years (Duke). Scientists can identify 450 substances in an apple. However, they still do not know enough about each of these to know how one interacts with the other 449 or how much each person may need and for what reason. Furthermore, as new phytochemicals are being discovered within foods every year, science can never truly ever say that they know what the body needs or even be able to accurately measure those needs.

Supplements can also cause harm to the body. These pills or additives to food can interfere with medication, leach other minerals and vitamins from a person's body and even settle in the human body. People may think they are getting the right nutrition use this as an excuse to eat a hurried diet or people may purchase enriched foods rather than whole foods because they believe they are eating nutritional equivalents. Many people also believe that vitamins and minerals are safe and that they can consume them as often as they like. However the phytochemicals that the body needs interact and depend on each other. Every mineral and vitamin a person consumes needs another mineral or vitamin to be assimilated into the body.

So if a person takes an excess of one or two nutrients they do not need, they are at the same time depleting their body of nutrients it may need (Heinerman). Many vitamins and minerals need sodium and potassium to assimilate into the body. So by taking a multi-vitamin, one could actually deplete their body of potassium and sodium sources. Some vitamins and minerals, taken in excess may even cancel each other out or cancel the effects of prescription medication that a person may be taking.

The supplement that is the most commonly known to be dangerous to humans is the iron supplement. Common iron pills contain 60 - 300mg of iron, even though the recommended daily allowance (RDA) is 1.7 - 7.8mg for infants, 6.1 - 8.7mg for children, and 8.7 - 11.3mg for men (Balch). American foods are routinely fortified with iron; but depending ones' level of deficiency, only 15 - 45% of the iron is even utilized. A high phosphorus diet, poor digestion, ulcers, excessive use of antacids, and the consumption of coffee and tea can also cause iron deficiencies. However, people who believe they need more iron in their diet may simply have the problem of not being able to circulate the iron they do have stored in the body OR they may be lacking in vitamin C or other vitamins that iron needs to assimilate. For this reason most people actually have an excess of iron rather than a deficiency in their diet. Excess dietary iron can increase the risk of bacterial infection. Studies in South East Asia and in Africa reveal that even low doses of iron supplements can be harmful if one is not iron deficient. When iron supplements were given to the Somali and Masai people, their rates of infection increased - even though their iron deficiency was corrected.

Iron, in the form of pills, interferes with zinc absorption and actually aggravates a zinc deficiency. Drinking a glass of orange juice with a meal or eating a fruit that is high in vitamin C - such as kiwis, citrus or berries - can increase absorption however, any extra iron is initially stored in the liver, with excess amounts being stored in the pancreas, lungs, spleen and heart. These excess amounts build up and destroy the tissues of the storage organs. Iron can also lead to impotence in men and amenorrhea (abnormal suppression or absence of menses) in young women. Women with chronic candida or herpes are susceptible to iron deficiencies and those who have cancer or rheumatoid arthritis have difficulty assimilating iron as well. People with sickle cell anemia, thalassemia or hemochromatosis should not take iron and it should be used carefully during pregnancy. Humans should especially avoid synthetic iron (ferrous sulfate) and use only organic iron and comprehensive lab tests should be performed before taking any supplements and any ingestion of iron should be done under the supervision of a doctor (Heinerman).

Although iron is famous for its dangers, there are many other vitamins that can be dangerous when taken in excess. Excess vitamin A or E can cause the blood to thin and excess vitamin C can cause cancer cells to multiply. Multivitamins are also one of the most harmful supplements available on the market today. Taking multiple vitamins can actually deplete the body of nutrients. Taking a pre-packaged multi-vitamin, no matter how high the quality is akin to following a "universal diet." Each person's nutrient needs are personal and chances are that one multi-vitamin will not fit everyone's needs. When this occurs, rather than help a person, the vitamin throws the body off balance.

Supplements do have a use in the medical field, however. In the hands of trained doctors, vitamins and minerals can actually provide intense emergency help to humans when used as a medical tool. Orthomolecular therapists have come up with precise ways to use vitamins and minerals in large doses to cure many hard to cure diseases from cancer to multiple sclerosis. However, the way in which they use vitamins is more akin to prescription medications than over-the counter usage. Dosages must be precise, must be monitored by a doctor and side effects are carefully scrutinized. The patient is then weaned off of the vitamin "medication" when they are healed (Hoffer).

Problems arise when studies stemming from such successes get re-written into laymen's language and become headlines like "Vitamin C Could Cure Cancer" The same articles usually forget to mention that people who were assisted in their cure by vitamin C were supervised by doctors and that heavy use of vitamin C could actually cause cancer cells to thrive. However, vitamins do have one advantage over prescription medications in that the chances of a fatal overdose are rarer. Vitamins themselves rarely cause death when taken in mega doses since a person's body usually eliminates the excess. Minerals, although less forgiving than vitamins (because they are stored in the body's bone and muscle tissue and can build up and cause toxicity), can only be overdosed when taken in very high amounts. This is in harsh contrast to drugs, where just a small overdose could kill or injure a person.

Scientists have recently been looking into the limitations of vitamin therapy in the general market. The results of this research have cause some scientists to realize that the search for factory created food supplements is an endless quest These scientists have created a new kind of supplement made only from whole foods. This new kind of supplement has been promoted as the "new and improved multivitamin" because manufacturers take foods straight from nature itself, reduce them into a pill and provide people with an easy way to consume more nutrients – even the ones that man may not be aware of. However, even these new pills pose a number of issues. The main problem with promoting such substances as nutrient supplements is that one needs to take so much of the substance to gain benefit that they become financially dependant on the company manufacturing them. Beyond this, promoting such substances as whole foods is misleading. The definition of a whole food is a food that has come straight from nature without any processing. Once a food is picked, sits for some time on a shelf, is chilled or boiled, dried, ground, packaged, and then shipped in the mail it is no longer a whole food (Hienerman). There are many phytochemicals that are lost in the process of sitting. More are lost as the food is chilled or steamed and even more are lost in the drying process. Packaging eliminates some more and by the time the "whole food" supplement arrives at one's door it is no longer a whole food. It is not as dangerous as synthetic supplements can be. However, it is ultimately an imperfect substitute for a healthy diet and a very cost-inefficient method of becoming healthier.

Ultimately whole foods as they are found in nature are the way to good health. Man does not need to search for a better way to stay healthy, but rather needs to become more acquainted with the healthy foods that are already provided to him and the best ways in which to combine and prepare these foods. It is surprising how many people can recite the virtues of vitamin C or taking a daily multivitamin but do not know why brown rice is better than white rice, why fresh juices are better than packaged ones or why it is best to eat foods in season to maintain optimum health. Supplements can be used to heal, but they should be used as close to their natural form as possible.

Assignment for Sections Four and Five

After reading chapters three, four and five choose a program for yourself and one other person you know. Choose a diet suitable for each "client" (yourself and the other person), as well as vitamins to supplement this diet. Please give at least five reasons you have made the choices in diet and vitamins that you made.

~Section Six: The Kitchen Pharmacy~

This book may look like "just a list" but it represents years of research and testing by The BEarth Institute. All the following folk remedies have been tested by The BEarth Institute instructors, students and clients. In addition they have all been cross-referenced in historical herb books, world traditions, and folk medicine. These healing foods have been well tested! We "threw out" numerous remedies we had found over the years that either were: very slow to work, did not work in all cases, were difficult to make or administer, or were too expensive and complex. This is what we were left with.

Acute Cures

Asthma - Apples, Garlic Syrup (see recipe below)⬚

Canker Sore- dip your finger in water and then mustard powder. Hold it to the canker sore for 5 minutes three times a day and it will be gone in 48 hours and not the three weeks it may take otherwise.⬚

Constipation - rub the abdomen in a clockwise motion with olive oil for 5-10 minutes, drink a glass of cold water with lemon first thing in the morning, eat a few figs and a ripe banana, sprinkle oat bran in your food, eat 1/8 cup of raw rice each morning, drink a glass of water with a TBS. of cornmeal in it each morning, drink aloe vera upon waking and before bed, Drink a glass of orange juice or grapefruit juice first thing in the morning, eat apples often, overnight soak six prunes in water, in the morning eat the prunes and drink the water, Constipation Candy: process 1/2 lb. of prunes, 1/2 lb. of raisins, 1/2 lb. of figs, 1/2 lb. of apricots and combine with 1/2 cup of oat bran or wheat bran. Roll into balls.⬚

Cold Sores- hold ice to the sore as much as you can throughout the day. It will go away in 48 hours. Or use yogurt or buttermilk, or aloe vera gel and do the same thing.⬚

Colds - at the onset grate some fresh ginger and heat it in warm water. Drink a few times a day, drink 10-20 drops of Tabasco sauce in water a few times a day,⬚

Cough - Make a hole in a big onion, fill it with honey and roast it. Drink the syrup as a cough syrup. Combine 1 tsp. of lemon with 1 tsp. of raw honey and sip this every half hour until the cough goes away. Garlic Cough Syrup: Peel and mince 8 cloves. Put them in a jar with a cup of raw honey. Let this stand for two hours. Take a tsp. at a time. Cough-Away Tea: Grate half an ounce of ginger into a cup of boiling water and let it sit. While it is sitting shell three walnuts. Drink the tea and walnuts together (swallow the grated ginger without chewing) you should wake up with no cough or phlegm. Thyme tea. Rub garlic on the bottom of the feet.⬚

Diarrhea - To destroy the harmful bacteria take a tbs. of ACV in water before each meal time, Drink a heaping tsp. of cornstarch in a glass of water. Repeat in 2-3 hours if this did not work the first time. or use 1 tsp. of carob powder in a glass of water. Grate an apple and let it sit until it turns brown. (This oxidizes⬚into what is used in many over the counter cough remedies). Sprinkle 1/4 tsp. of cinnamon on it and eat it. Mash a banana and carob together to make a carob pudding. Eat it.⬚

Earache - puncture a garlic clove and squeeze it into your ear. Put a cotton ball over your ear. This relieves pain as well as kills infection. If you get infections to often then prevent them by putting a few drops of jojoba or mineral oil in your ear once a month to keep the wax cleared out.

Eczema - eat one TBS. blackstrap molasses daily. eat one raw potato a day (you can juice this and mix it with apple juice). Eat a few tsp. of watercress each day. Drink aloe vera juice after each meal (one ounce).⬚

Fatigue - thump your thymus glands like a gorilla for about one minute, or press your knees together tightly for two minutes, Eat some sunflower seeds. Drink rosemary lemonade, Energy drink - 6 oz. un sweetend cranberry juice, 2 oz. orange juice, 1 lime, ice and water.⬚

Gas - take a tsp. of aloe vera at every meal time. Cut four slices off of a fresh ginger root and drop it in a mug of boiled water. Let steep for five minutes and drink after any gas-causing meal. When you cook beans always have greens with them. Or add a cut up potato while cooking beans (you can discard the potato later). Or after eating beans eat watermelon.⬚

Headache - Swing your arms like the "windmill". This increases circulation to the arms and lessens the circulation to the head and reduces pain. Alternatively, try increasing circulation to the area by rubbing your shoulders and loosening up any tenseness. Dip a bandanna in vinegar and wrap it around your head. Wear it until the headache goes away. OR just tie the bandanna tightly around your head over the eyebrows OR just use the ACV. Mix 2 TBS. ACV with 2 tsp. of honey in a glass of water and drink slowly, results within a half hour. For a Migraine : put your feet in a basin of hot water and and ice pack on the back of your neck. eat 12 raw almonds if you are not allergic,⬚

Heartburn - Mix 2 TBS. of olive oil and an egg white and drink it down. Take some coffee grounds and hold them in your mouth to soak them with your saliva then spit them out. Put 2 iceberg lettuce leaves with 6 oz. of water and blend. Drink the mixture.⬚

Itching - soak a cloth in milk and put it over the itch. Rub sea salt on the area after wetting it.

Insomnia - Chop a yellow onion and put it in a jar by your bed. Whiff it and think happy thoughts for fifteen minutes. You should be sleeping by then. Eat pumpkin at your evening meal s a side dish or desert. Stuff a little pillow with celery seeds and sleep near or on it.⬚

Hives - Mix 1 ounce of white vinegar with three ounces of cornstarch and dab the hives.

Leg Cramps - This may seem strange but it works! Take a piece of stainless steel or silver spoon and put it by your bed. When you wake with a cramp, put the silverware on top of it and it will un cramp.⬚

Libido - Halva, Eat sunflower seeds, any hot spices. Make a cardamom cinnamon tea with milk.

Motion Sickness - Smell a green apple, suck on a lemon, drink ginger ale or ginger tea, eat two or three olives, eat a bowl of vegetable soup with 1/4-1/2 tsp. of cayenne pepper in it.

Neuralgia - Massage fresh lemon juice on the painful areas. bake a potato, when it cools off, cut it in half and place the white side down on the painful areas.

Nausea - homemade ginger ale.

Sinus attack - take some raw honey and chew the wax for a few minutes. It will usually stop sinus attacks. Dissolve 1 tsp. salt (sea salt is best) in one cup warm spring or distilled water. With your hands or medicine dropper inhale this through the nose and spit it out your mouth. This clears up most anything. Can be used daily. You get used to it.

Sore throat - take a TBS. of honey and squeeze half and lemon into it. Drink this every half hour. Mix two tsp. ACV in a glass of water. Drink a bit and gargle with it, drink some and gargle with some and spit, then drink some and gargle with the next mouthful. Keep alternating until there is no liquid left. Drink grapefruit juice. Eat fresh pineapple.

Chronic Cures

Allergy Fighter - Carrot-Celery Juice - After Chlorine exposure, for anti-allergy cures *Bed wetting* - Chew on Cinnamon bark during the day and a spoon of raw honey at night.

Anti-Allergenic Stuffed animals - put them in the freezer once a week for 24 hours to kill the dust mites.

Gallstones / Sluggish Gallbladder or Liver - Lie down on the floor or bed and slowly sip 1/2 cup of warm olive oil (with lemon or grapefruit juice if you want for added effect). You may experience discomfort, but the gallstones should pass in 48 hours. Alternatively you could take 2 TBS. of live oil in a glass of grapefruit juice daily every morning. Increase the amount gradually until you are up to 1/4 cup of juice. By the end of the month your problem will be gone.

Hair Loss - Put 2 ounces of barley with 6 cups of water. Boil down to half. Drink this liquid. Wash your hair with sage tea daily. Ginger Grow-Back remedy: Grate a ginger and spread it on the bald area. Cover your head with a shower cap for a half hour before shampooing. Do this daily.

Kidney Problems - Watermelon seed tea (1tsp. of watermelon seeds in boiling water. Let steep for ten minutes). Parsley -carrot juice.

Ulcers - start with 1/8 tsp. of cayenne pepper in a glass of water and work up to 1/4 tsp. twice a day. It takes some getting used to but it works and also dulls the pain. One tablespoon of aloe vera after each meal. Raw cabbage juice twice a day (1/2 cup). Barley water three times a day.

Warts - put on some ACV a few times a day,. When it dries brush it with baking soda. Do this until the wart disappears. Put raw eggplant on it overnight, held on with a band aid

Pregnancy - For prevention of miscarriage drink two cups of sage tea daily for the first three months. Rub sesame oil or olive oil on your belly daily to prevent stretch marks.⬚Do the same rub for the opening of the vagina to prevent tears.⬚Starting in the third month eat onions and garlic daily for an easier birth and more stamina.

Morning sickness - to prevent eat a cup of dark greens with every meal.

Weight Control - Drink tomato juice before you eat⬚1 TBS. of ACV and 1 TBS. of honey in a glass of water and drink it before you eat Rinse your mouth with baking soda to suppress a sugar urge/sweet tooth.

Mosquito repellent - Rub ACV in yourself or exposed areas or spray it on. Eat lots of garlic, eat a raw onion or two, rub sprigs of parsley on your exposed skin.⬚

Fruit and vegetable wash - Fill a basin with cold water, the juice of one lemon and 4 TBS. of salt. This makes a weak form of hydrochloric acid. You can also fill a sink with water, pour in a half cup of vinegar and 1/8th cup baking soda (optional) and wait for it to fizz. Veggies soak five-ten minutes. Fruits soak 2 .

For High blood pressure eat - Kiwi, Bananas, green leafy vegetables, oranges ,potatoes with peel, sunflower seeds.⬚

For Hair Loss Eat - Cabbage, Brussel Sprouts ,Kale, Watercress, Cauliflower, Raspberries, Cranberries, Barley.

High Cholesterol eat - olive oil - no other oil, butter or oil or butter substitute,⬚brussel sprouts and cabbage several times a week, raw garlic in salads or dressing⬚1/2 cup of beans a day, raw carrots - eat a few a day, broccoli, onions, 1/2 cup of oat bran a day, oat meal, eggplant rids the body of cholesterol before it can be absorbed by the body - so enjoy your musakka!, grapefruit, apples.

Personal Care Products

Dandruff Shampoo - Cut a leaf the night before you shampoo. Rub the gel in your hair and sleep with a bandanna on. In the morning lather up the aloe and wash your hair. Or saturate your hair with ACV and wait one hour. rinse. Do this twice a week until the dandruff clears.⬚Wrinkle remover - Do this once in the morning and once before sleeping: Put two slices of lemon in a WOODEN bowl. Heat some half and half and add it to cover the lemons. For oily skin use 3 lemons, for dry skin use 1 lemon and double the half and half. Let this sit for three hours.. Strain and massage the liquid into your face and neck with your middle three fingertips working upwards and outwards in a small circular motions. Let it dry then remove with a little water and olive oil after fifteen minutes.

Deodorant - Baking soda: Underarm deodorant when combined with cornstarch or rice starch and/or powdered herbs (like sage). Also good for toothpaste when mixed with sea salt.□

Deep Conditioning - Ripe banana: Thank goodness you can stop making banana bread. Instead rub this on your hair , wrap your hair in a towel for an hour and wash. Instant and wonderful conditioner!

Split ends - Rub 1/2 cup of olive oil in your hair, then wash with shampoo mixed with one egg yolk, then rinse with apple cider vinegar and water. Good split end cure!□Facials - rub crushed honeydew melon on your face to condition it. Mix 2 TBS.> light cream of yogurt with honey and rub on your face to moisturize and condition. For dry skin, beat two egg yolks and smear them on your face. Lie on a slant board or with feet elevated while you relax. Do not talk. Wash off after 20 minutes. For oily skin use egg whites.

Hair spray: - I hate the stuff so this natural one is a life saver! Take two large lemons and chunk them. Put them in an enamel saucepan. Add two cups of water and bring to a boil. Simmer for twenty minutes. Store in the refrigerator or add a preservative of alcohol to preserve it.

Deodorant: - Half apple cider vinegar and water sprayed under the arms is a good deodorant.

Suntan Lotion - 1/2 ACV and 1/2 olive oil protects the skin from burning and chapping.

Dandruff Prevention - Slathering Yoghurt on your hair as a prewash kills the candida bacteria that create many dandruff problems.

Recipes

Apple Cider Vinegar Tonic

2 tsp. RAW honey□2 tsp. Apple Cider Vinegar 8 oz. of water

Drink before every meal , upon rising and at bedtime

This "tonic" is said to...□cure arthritis and other pains.□assist in weight loss by helping fat absorption and suppressing appetite, stop the hiccups.□stop leg cramps.□improve memory, cure morning sickness when taken first thing in the morning. Double the dose for a sinusitis relief.□eases Gas.□eases upset stomach.

Other uses for Apple Cider Vinegar:□**Sprinkle a pillow with ACV to alleviate a cough.□**To banish dandruff rinse hair with 1/2 cup ACV in 2 cups of water after each shampoo until you get results (usually three shampoos).□**Dilute and put a few drops in your ear to prevent "swimmers ear".□**Add a TBS. of ACV to warm water and gargle as a mouthwash or for a sore throat.□**Dab it on your forehead while resting to alleviate headache.□**Start each day with a glass of water with 4 tsp. ACV, black strap molasses and honey for a rich, thick and not gray head of hair your whole life□**Take 1 tsp. three times a day in apple cider for a heart tonic to prevent heart attacks. **Sore throat rememdy:1/2 cup ACV, 1/2 cup water, 1 tsp. cayenne pepper, 3 TBS. honey. Sip occasionally throughout the day. Sudanese Cayenne "Shatta" Squeeze one lime into a bowl. Mix in enough very hot cayenne pepper to make a paste. Add a pinch of salt. At meal times dip bread in this, add it to your soup or make it thinner and pour it over vegetables. This shatta is said to: prevent heart attacks (for an actual attack take two capsules). reduce risk of stroke (for actual stroke take 2 capsules). take away arthritis pain. reduce asthma attacks and bronchitis. stop a runny nose. Put the sauce in a glass of water (2 tsp.) a drink it.

Garlic Syrup

Take 1/2 pound peeled garlic buds. Add equal amounts apple cider vinegar and distilled water to cover the buds. Add later 1/2 pint of glycerin and 1 1/2 pounds of honey. Put vinegar and garlic in a wide mouth jar and shake well. Let stand in a cool place four or five days, shaking each day. Add the glycerin, shake the jar and let stand one more day. Strain and blend in the honey.

This is good for: Give 1 tsp. of this tonic to a person having an asthma attack every 15 minutes until the spasm is controlled. Give 1 TBS. three times a day with meals for the following: deep coughs bronchitis high blood pressure circulation problems heart disease infections cancer bacterial infections, detoxification blood sugar problems digestive problems fights free radicals in the body from pollution really, everything....

Other uses for garlic: Rub the soles of the feet with it to prevent nightmares. Cook in vegetable soup to cure a cold fast or assist in recovery. Removes lice: mix ten tsp. of oil and ten cloves of minced garlic . Cover and leave for 36 hours. Strain, then massage it into the head and cover with a warm towel. Shampoo off after one hour. Heals Hemorrhoids: Peel a clove and insert it in the rectum overnight. This also expels pinworms and other worms. Acne: for acne, spots and ulcers, press crushed garlic to the area for a few minutes each day.

Honey Tonic Balls

1 cup tahini
1/2 cup honey
1 T. local bee pollen
1 T. black seed (ground or mashed with mortar and pestle)
1 TBS. Sunflower seeds (optional)

1 TBS. black sesame seeds (optional) Wheat or Oat bran or Muesli. Add any of the following: raisins, dry milk powder, powdered herbs, cayenne, cinnamon, oats, carob powder. Other uses for honey: Put on wounds to heal them. Put on a burn. Take 1-2 tsp. in water for stomach problems. Give a TBS. of honey to bed wetting child before bed (and restrict liquids for two hours before this. Have them brush their teeth afterwards too). Mix 1 tsp. honey in barley water. This stops diarrhea, opens obstructions of liver, kidney and bladder. General tonic.

Aloe Vera Juice

Massage the forehead with a mix of aloe and rosewater for a headache cure. Opens the liver obstructions and cures depression. Cures jaundice Relieves side effects of many drugs. Apply for an acne cure Can lower blood pressure Help stomach burning Put it on burns Prevents asthma when taken after each meal. Constipation cure - take upon rising and before bed

Constipation Candy

Process 1/2 lb. of prunes, 1/2 lb. of raisins, 1/2 lb. of figs, 1/2 lb. of apricots and combine with 1/2 cup of oat bran or wheat bran. Roll into balls and eat a couple daily.

Homemade Halva

Grind 1 cup of sesame seeds. Mix with raw honey until it makes a firm dough. Eat it like candy. Very high in calcium. This is in fact better than taking a calcium and vitamin E supplement daily!

Homemade Ginger Ale

Take 2 cups fresh ginger root, sliced but not peeled. Put in 4 cups of water. Simmer on low for half an hour. Strain. Add one half cup of maple syrup or honey. Cool and store in the fridge for six months. Add to hot water to make tea or fizzy water to make ginger ale.

Barley Water (Talbiyah)

Put 1 cup of barley with 6 cups of water. Boil down to half. Drink this liquid. Use crushed barley. This is more effective. Stimulates bowel movements. Solves most digestive problems. Quenches the thirst Lowers a temperature. Soothes the spirit and relieves depression. Nourishes an undernourished body.

Tonic Salad Dressing

1/2 cup ACV
4 TBS. raw honey
4 raw garlic cloves, crushed
1/2 tsp. cayenne pepper (optional)
1/8 cup olive oil

Congee 1 cup of rice 6 cups of water. Simmer the rice and water for 4-6 hours together with: Aduki bean for edema and gout Carrot to aid in digestion Chicken for wasting illness and recovery Mung bean for relieving fever and cooling a person Salted onion to lubricate the muscles Purslane for detoxification, rheumatism and swelling. Sesame seed : for rheumatism Cook these into the congee in the last hour. Add spices and salt as needed.

Acidophilis Supplement-Rejuvelac

2 cups wheat berries
1 quart of water

Soak 2 cups of wheat berries for one day. Discard the water. Rinse the berries and soak them again in a jar covered with a sprout screen or cloth. Let stand for two days. Pour off the rejuvelac. Add one more quart of water to the wheat berries. After one day pour off the second batch. You can keep this going for several weeks. Drink this as a natural acidophilis supplement. A cup a day is good.

Seed Yogurt Protein and acidophilis supplement 1 cup of sesame seeds or sunflower seeds, soaked overnight (discard the soaking water in the morning) 1 cup rejuvelac or water 1/2 tsp. soy sauce or miso Blend seeds at a high speed. Slowly pour in the liquid and soy sauce until creamy. Add some previously made seed yogurt if you have it to speed fermentation. Set in a warm place and cover (do not seal). Let ferment 6-10 hours then refrigerate.

Lemons

Lemons are tonic, aid in digestion, have anti-infection action, clean the skin, tone the heart, decongest the liver and kill bacteria (this may be why in the Middle East they squeeze lemon over the fresh salad).

Uses for lemon Digestive aid/liver decongestant: The juice of one lemon in water taken first thing in the morning increases digestive juices, tones the system and cleanses the liver. It also helps constipation. Take a glass of cold water first thing in the morning. Follow this with a glass of lemon and water. Blood Purifier: Drink lots of lemonade (lemon water or lemon water with stevia or honey - no sugar!) to cleanse the skin of boils, eczema and other skin problems). Skin Cleanser: Rub lemon on the skin to eliminate blackheads and acne. Coughs: Wash the lemon, put the uncut edge in a dish of honey and a handful of cloves. Soak the lemon and honey overnight. Cut the lemon in half and squeeze all the juice in the honey. Use this liquid in small doses throughout the day. Heart and circulation problems: take lemon water 3 times a day to strengthen the heart & blood vessels. Water purifier: If you are questioning the purity of your water, a lemon squeezed into it will kill many things and most bacteria. Fever reducer: lemon water or lemon added to barley water (see above) revive a sick person and reduce the fever. Pains: Rub lemons on the skin for rheumatism pains, arthritis and other pains. Also drink two - three glasses internally daily. Kidney and Bladder Infection: Drink lemon water daily to clear these.

Healing Properties of Common Culinary Herbs

THYME: Thyme is used in feminine hygiene douches, Vicks Vapo-rub, ear drops and Listerine mouthwash, and anti-fungal cremes⬚Woman's Herb for Pain in Menses, All Uterine Problems (but not during pregnancy) - infusion three times a day⬚Gastric Problems of all sorts - infusion three times a day⬚Bad Breath - gargle infusion⬚Wind/ Gas - infusion three times a day⬚Fever - infusion taken in 1/4 cup portions every ten minutes for two hours (adult)⬚Headache - infusion four times a day. You can also take it as for a fever⬚Antiseptic Action for Eczema, Ringworm, Psoriasis, Parasitic Infections, Burns - infusion soaked in a cloth and applied to area.⬚Insect Repellent - infusion put in a bottle and sprayed on skin or fresh dried herbs hung or spread on problem area⬚Stomach Ache - infusion three times a day⬚Whooping Cough - 3-5 cups a day (adult)⬚Sore Throat - gargle with and drink infusion three times a day⬚Lung Tonic - infusion three times a day⬚Poultice for Boils, Sciatic Pain, or Swellings - make a paste with water and dried leaves. Apply to area and cover with a cheesecloth and then a cotton or wool rag. Leave on with pressure for half hour.⬚Deodorant - spray on infusion and drink three cups a day

SAGE: ⬚An English proverb says "why should a man die while sage grows in his garden?" Depression - drink infusion with a clove to lift depression. Up to four cups a day.⬚Breath Freshener - rub the leaves across your teeth⬚Fever - Add 10 cups of the infusion to bathwater, rub on the body and drink with lemon and honey in 1/4 cup portions over the course of two hours every 15 minutes. (adult)⬚Antiseptic - chew sage leaves to cleanse your system, Use the tea to clean cutting boards, the children's room after a sickness, the bathroom counter, etc...⬚Gargle - use the infusion as a gargle⬚Sleep - Drink alone or with peppermint and chamomile to induce sleep (in children...)⬚Sore throat - drink and gargle with infusion⬚Stomach Trouble - drink 3 cups of the COLD infusion daily⬚Flu - drink 4 cups of infusion a day.⬚Varicose Veins - apply sage compress to the legs and take sage (infused tea) footbaths daily. Wounds and Old Sores - wash with infusion

MINT: Arthritis or Rheumatism - soak a cloth in the infusion and apply to skin⬚Digestive Aid - infusion after meals⬚Headache (sinus headache or digestion related headaches) - infusion four times a day. Muscle Spasms/ cramps - apply infusion externally, drink three times a day. Sinus Problems - apply a peppermint pack to the nasal area, drink the infusion four times a day.

PARSLEY: ⬚Diuretic - juice as 1/4 of the cup of fresh juice - remaining of the cup can be any juice like apple, or carrot or make as an infusion three times a day⬚Breath Freshener - Chew on the fresh leaves⬚CLOVES⬚Chew on a clove to numb toothache and get fresh breath. Also is an antiseptic for sore and damaged gums. When the oil has been infused twice it is ready to use in SMALL PORTIONS (a Q- tip applied to the gums).⬚Sleep Aid - Add a few cloves to boiling water and simmer for three minutes. Add milk or soy milk and honey and zzzz.......⬚Depression - Make the tea as above three times a day WITH MEALS so you don't fall asleep or without the milk.⬚Nausea Aid - Make tea as above to help all digestive problems, especially nausea and weak digestion or desire to eat.⬚Paper Cuts or Minor Cuts - Dip your wet finger in a bowl of powdered cloves. The anesthetic action will make the pain disappear!

CINNAMON: Arthritis or Rheumatism - soak a cloth in the decoction and apply to joints⏺Circulation - take three cups of the decoction for bad circulation or chills⏺Diarrhea - use the decoction three times a day⏺Flu Preventative - Make a cinnamon bark decoction and take three times a day with honey. Morning Sickness - Infuse the bruised bark with any other tea about an hour before bedtime.. You can also make a decoction with the bark and take 1 tsp. at a time before meals to relieve nausea.⏺Anti-nausea formula - 3 small thin sticks of cinnamon bark, 8 cardamom seeds, 1 TBS. (or one medium) nutmeg. Grind this all together in a grinder. Place it in a jar and label "anti-nausea". Use 1/4 tsp. to one cup of water for an adult. Prepare as an infusion. Use a pinch to cooled tea for a child.⏺Negativity - Ever heard of those polarizers that absorb negative energy? Cinnamon Bark in your pocket does the same thing.⏺Cramps - Make a decoction alone or with other herbs for menstrual cramps.

Instructions on Preparation of Remedies

Hot Infusion⏺

30g of dried herb (1 ounce or 2 TBS.)⏺
500ml of water (2 cups)⏺

1. Boil the water
2. Pour the water over the herb
3. Let sit 20 minutes
4. Strain the herbs.
5. Drink one cup three times a day for adults⏺
6. Strained herbal tea can be stored in a stainless steel thermos all day or in a glass jar or pitcher (with lid) in the refrigerator up to three days

Cold Infusion⏺

30g of dried herb (1 ounce or 2 TBS.)⏺
500ml of water (2 cups)⏺

1. Pour water over herbs in a pitcher with lid.⏺
2. Leave to sit all night and strain and store in the morning.

Decoction⏺30g of dried herb (1 ounce or 2 TBS.)⏺750ml of water boiled down to 500ml (3 cups boiled down to 2 cups)⏺1. Place the herbs in a stainless steel saucepan or glass pan⏺2. Add cold water⏺3. Bring herbs to a boil, then simmer for about 1 hour until volume is reduced by 1/3 and the water now measures about 500ml (you can approximate this and add more water later to bring it up to 500ml if you have to).⏺4. Strain herbs out through a muslin cloth to be able to squeeze all the juice out of them. Portions: Same guidelines as above**

Syrup

Make a quadruple strength decoction (Simmer down to 1/2 cup instead of two)125ml (1/2 cup) of decoction (see above)Add 125ml (1/2 cup) of honey or vegetable glycerine**and heat and stir together until honey is dissolved (5 minutes). Cool and store in a glass corked bottle in the refrigerator up to 3 months. Dose for adults is 2 TBS. 3 times a day. For children: 1-2 Tsp. 3 times a day (see hcp). **vegetable glycerine can be found at pharmacies. Make sure it is the quality for consumption. This is a little better than honey to use so try to find some if you can. Although honey still is effective.

Cooking With Herbal Teas

Most people think of herbal teas as something to drink, but you can also enjoy the benefits of herbal teas by using them in your cooking. Besides enjoying the same benefits you would by drinking a cup of tea, you can also create wonderful , unusual and special meals and deserts using herbal teas. These meals are perfect for special occasions or as a special treat for your family. Following are some basic directions for using herbal teas in cooking:

Follow these rules to get the maximum benefit out of your herbal tea dishes:1. Don't microwave your food that you have or will cook with the tea. Use the stove.2. Do not bake herbal tea dishes3. Try to choose dishes that have a minimal cooking time, so as to minimize the amount of cooking the teas go through. The more you cook or bake them, the less effective the therapeutic benefits, although the flavor will still be delightful.4. Use only fresh dried or fresh herbal teas. Do not use tea bags or boxed teas if you expect any therapeutic benefits from your dishes. You can get fresh teas from Mountain Rose Herbs and Frontier Herbs.

Herbal Soup

General directions: Make your favorite soup. One half hour before it is finished put a two TBS of your herbal tea in a boqui garni bag and continue to simmer your soup. Good choices for soup depending on what kind you are making are: Try to use a combination of at least three from each list.

Nourishing herbs: nettles, alfalfa, red clover, horsetail, oatstraw, hops, & parsley.Healing herbs traditional flavor: thyme, sage, rosemary, basilHealing herbs flowers & sweet flavor: calendula, cinnamon, lemon balm, raspberry leaf, & dandelion, cardamom, anise.

Herbal Pudding

General directions: Make an herbal infused milk by putting 1/8 cup of fresh dried herbs into 4-6 cups of milk in a jug overnight. In the morning strain the herbs out and either make your own favorite homemade pudding recipe or add a box of instant pudding mix and let set. Choose your herbs and pudding flavor carefully. Mint Chocolate is nice for children and Rose Petal Vanilla is a wonderful gourmet pudding for guests, but disliked by many children. Before serving top the pudding with some leaves of the herbs you used (mint leaves or rose petals, etc.....) for a final touch. Some suggested combinations: Rose petal, vanilla⬛chocolate mint,⬛lemon balm mint, or lemon balm vanilla, cinnamon apple,⬛calendula & lavender, vanilla anise-fennel, vanilla⬛marshmallow butterscotch,⬛chamomile vanilla.

Herbal Punch

Add 1/4 cup of fresh dried herbs to bottled, canned or mixed-up frozen or homemade punch. Let sit overnight and in the morning strain out the herbs. Serve! Some of my favorite combinations include:⬛Alertness Drink- Rosemary & lemonade

Energy Drink- Mint, nettles, alfalfa & lemonade⬛Slumber Punch - Hibiscus or berry punch with chamomile & rose petals⬛Nourishing Punch - Nettles, oat straw, alfalfa, red raspberry leaf and cranberry juice Pregnancy Punch - Orange juice, red raspberry leaf, nettles, oat straw, and spearmint Nursing Punch - Fennel, anise and apple cider

Herbal Muffins

Use herbal tea or infused milk instead of milk in your favorite muffin recipe. Bake and mix as directed. You can even used boxed muffins for this. Some good ideas are: cinnamon pumpkin muffins, mint orange muffins,⬛hibiscus blueberry muffins, lemon balm poppy seed muffins

Herbal Salad Dressing/ Sauce

Make or buy your favorite salad dressing, put it in a jug or jar and put 1/8-1/4 cup of herbs in the jar. Shake well and return to the refrigerator. Do this for three days. On the third day, strain out the herbs and use. Some good combinations are:⬛Healing dressing: Echinacea root and creamy dressing. Perky dressing: Nettles, alfalfa, red clover and vinaigrette

Perky Herbal Salad Dressing

1/3 cup balsamic or apple cider vinegar
1/3 cup olive oil
1 TBS Dijon mustard
1 tsp. salt
1 tsp. garlic
1 TBS nettles
1 TBS alfalfa
1 TBS red clover

Mix all ingredients together. Store in refrigerator for three days, shaking once or twice a day. At the end of three days strain out the herbs & use.

Healing Vegetable Herb Soup

4 cups of soup stock or water
4 cups of chopped potatoes, carrots, onions, green beans, & zucchini
4 TBS tomato paste
2 tsp. salt
1 TBS thyme, rosemary & sage in a bouquet garni bag.

Cook vegetables and stock with salt for 15 minutes. Add herbs. Cook for 15-30 minutes more. Add tomato paste & serve.

Relaxing Pudding

2 C. of milk infused with rose petals
3 T. Honey
3 TBS cornstarch
2 eggs - well beaten
1 T vanilla

Combine milk, honey and starch. Cook for 3 minutes over a slow burner. Beat in eggs and together 3 more minutes stirring constantly. Add vanilla & cool.

Other wild ideas: Feeling creative? You can use your infused milk anywhere even in such unusual places such as pancakes, milk shakes, homemade ice-cream, homemade cheeses & yogurts, pies, cakes and more! Here are some more ideas:

Ayurvedic Stew

1/2 tsp. olive oil
3/4 tsp. whole cumin seed
3/4 tsp. ground coriander
1/2 cup brown rice - cooked
1/2 cup mung beans -cooked

4 cups turmeric tea (take 4 tsp. of turmeric powder and pour 4 cups of boiled water over it. Strain out the herbs after 20 minutes OR preferably take 8 of the roots and simmer them in 4 cups of water for 20 minutes).

Try to find whole turmeric instead of powdered, but powdered will also do. This soup is a strengthening soup, helps in pain relief, regulates menses, decongest the liver, is antiseptic, kills bacteria and molds and aids in getting rid of yeast infections, relieves uterine spasms during period, assists digestive system and strengthens the reproductive system. The soup as a whole balances the energies of the body and is a tonic food. It soothes respiratory ailments, purifies the blood, and aids in relief of arthritis.

Vegetable Strengthening Soup

1/2 pound squash
2 carrots, sliced
1 large onion, sliced
1 leek, sliced
2 cloves garlic, peeled
1/2 cup fresh parsley
1/2 cup celery, chopped

Steam all of the above and tip into a blender and puree. You will have two cups of puree. Mix this puree with 1 cup of the water (the same water used to steam the vegetables!!!). Add: 1 tsp. reduced sodium soy sauce, 1 tsp. salt and 2 cups of strong rosemary tea (put 4 tsp. of rosemary leaves (not powdered) in a pan and pour boiling water over it. Let sit twenty minutes, then strain out the herbs. You will have 2 cups of strong rosemary tea). Blend all this together and heat.

This soup will wake you up and provide multiple vitamins and minerals. It aids memory, restores heath in long term illnesses, prevents disease, relieves all kinds of headaches and muscle spasms, relieves pain, increases alertness, stimulates circulation and the nervous system to relieve pain and depression. Aids arthritis and fatigue.

Peppermint Grapefruit punch

Make 2 cups of strong peppermint tea by pouring 2 cups of boiling water over 4 tsp. of peppermint. Strain out the herbs and chill this tea. When chilled add 1 cup of fresh grapefruit juice and 1 cup of Perrier (sparkling water). Drink this as a refresher AFTER MEALS. This drink will aid digestion, ease nausea, is cooling and acts as a tonic for the lungs. It will increase circulation, assist the sinuses and relieve headaches and fatigue.

Rosemary Soup

2 tsp. olive oil
3 large onions, thinly sliced
2 leeks, rinsed, trimmed and sliced
2 shallots, thinly sliced
2 cloves garlic, thinly sliced
1 bay leaf
4 cups rosemary tea (pour 4 cups of water over 4 tsp. rosemary and let steep for 20 minutes. Pour out the herbs)
1 tsp. salt
1 tsp. low sodium soy sauce
6 TBS. REAL parmesan cheese, grated.

Heat olive oil, add onions, leeks, shallots and garlic and bay leaf and sauté until tender (15 min). Discard the bay leaf. Add the rosemary tea , swirl in the cheese and serve the soup.

This soup will restore strength to the body, it increases circulation and brings warmth to the body, it detoxifies the body, reduces cholesterol, aids against flus, and aids against hypertension and diabetes. This soup will wake you up and provide multiple anti-oxidants to your system. It aids memory, restores heath in long term illnesses, prevents disease, relieves all kinds of headaches and muscle spasms, relieves pain, increases alertness, stimulates circulation and the nervous system to relieve pain and depression. Aids arthritis and fatigue. Some added benefits of this soup are that it protects against some cancers and provides some significant amounts of potassium and natural sodium to the body to aid in allergy relief.

Ginger & Cinnamon Smoothie

1 cup of yogurt (plain)
2 TBS. molasses (mild)
1 TBS. honey
1 tsp. vanilla
1 TBS. sesame seeds
1 TBS. sunflower seeds
1 tsp. Green Magma
1 cup of strong ginger-cinnamon tea (simmer 2 dried ginger roots and 2 cinnamon bark sticks in 1 cup of water for 20 minutes, then strain out the herbs)
Fresh pineapple or mango

Blend all this together in the blender.

This drink provides protein, iron, calcium, zinc, vitamin E, multiple vitamins and minerals, potassium and phosphorus. This is VERY high in calcium. This drink provides energy, aids in digestion and relieves nausea. It aids circulation and stimulates the body, thus relieving fatigue.It relieves cramps and spasms during the menses, and warms the stomach and increases desire for food in those who have bad appetite. It raises the vitality of the body, helps against rheumatism, stimulates all the vital functions of the body, aids against all sinus and/or congestive problems.

Tahini Herb Balls

1 cup tahini
1/2 cup honey (raw)
1 T. local bee pollen and royal jelly (you can buy honey with this mixed in already)
1 T. black seed (mashed with mortar and pestle)
1 TBS. Sunflower seeds (optional)
1 TBS. black sesame seeds (optional)
Cinnamon, powdered - 3 tsp.
Ginger, powdered - 3 tsp.
Green Magma - 3 tsp.
Oats and muesli - enough to make a firm dough.

Roll into 36 balls and take as snacks. No more than 6 a day.

This herb balls provide protein, iron, calcium, zinc, vitamin E, vitamin B multiple B's , multiple vitamins and minerals, potassium and phosphorus. This is VERY high in calcium. These balls provide energy, aid in digestion and relieve nausea. They aid circulation and stimulate the body, thus relieving fatigue. They relieve cramps and spasms during the menses, and warms the stomach and increases desire for food in those who have bad appetite. It raises the vitality of the body, helps against rheumatism, stimulate all the vital functions of the body, aids against all sinus and/or congestive problems. It contains many herbs and foods that are considered "ultimate tonics" or "cure-alls"

Turmeric Omelet w/ parsley, coriander and garlic

1 tsp. olive oil▯
1 tsp. turmeric powder▯
1/4 cup parsley▯
2 cloves garlic, sliced▯
1/8 cup coriander▯
1/2 cup onions.▯

Sauté all the above and pour over it three eggs beaten in 1/4 cup of water. Cook until firm omelet style or scrambled eggs. This omelet is a strengthening soup, helps in pain relief, regulates menses, decongest the liver, is antiseptic, kills bacteria and molds and aids in getting rid of yeast infections, relieves uterine spasms during period, assists digestive system and strengthens the reproductive system. It provides multiple vitamins and minerals. It provides magnesium.

Spiced Barley

1 cup cooked barley▯
1/2 cup fenugreek

Cloves, cinnamon and cardamom tea. (make tea by taking one cardamom pod, 1 tsp. of helba, 3 cloves, and one cinnamon stick and simmering it in 1 cup of soy milk for 15 minutes. Save the rest of the tea).

Pour the soy milk tea over the rice and swirl in a pinch of honey. Eat. You can also use rice or almond milk if you are not supposed to drink soy. This is high in fiber and helps stabilize blood sugar levels. This "cereal" provides energy, aids in digestion and relieves nausea. It aids circulation and stimulates the body, thus relieving fatigue. It relieves cramps and spasms during the menses, and warms the stomach and increases desire for food in those who have bad appetite. It raises the vitality of the body, helps against rheumatism, stimulates all the vital functions of the body, aids against all sinus and/or congestive problems. It aids against parasites and yeast infections and is high in protein and potassium and magnesium.

Sleepytime shake

1/2 large banana
1/2 pink grapefruit, peeled, seeded and sectioned
1/2 cup oatmilk (take 2 TBS. of oats and cook in 1/2 cup of water until it is milky)
1 cup strong sleepy time tea (take 1 tsp. of sleepy time herbs and pour over them one cup of water. Let sit for 15 minutes, then strain out the herbs).

Blend all this together in the blender and drink.

Sleepytime Soup

1/2 pound squash
2 medium carrots
1 large onion
2 cloves garlic

Steam the above vegetables in 2 cups water. Puree the steamed vegetables and add to the steaming water. Add the following: 1 TBS. toasted fennel seeds (heat on high in a sauté pan for two minutes), 2 tsp. herbal sleepy tea or chamomile tea 1 tomato, chopped 1 tsp. soy sauce Stir and simmer for 10 minutes, blend again if needed. You can eat the herbs blended or not blended in the soup.

Sleepytime "ice cream"

2 cups chopped fresh pumpkin (or two cups canned pumpkin)
1/4 tsp. orange zest
1 tsp. vanilla extract
1/2 tsp. pumpkin pie spice
1/4 cup maple syrup or honey
2 cups yogurt (plain)

Cook pumpkin until soft in 2-4 cups of chamomile or sleepy blend tea (pour 4 cups of water over 4 tsp. of tea. Let sit for 15 minutes and then strain out the herbs). Blend in blender until smooth, add rest of ingredients. Pour into a shallow pan and put in the freezer. Every half hour stir the mixture until it is completely frozen. Put in a closed container and eat.

Assignment for Section Six

There are a number of "kitchen remedies" mentioned in this short "reference book" chapter. Please choose ten of the remedies you are most likely to use on this list and tell why you are most likely to use them. Please also choose ten remedies from this list you "wish you had used" at some time in the past year or two. Give reasons why.